PCOS Diet for the Newly Diagnosed

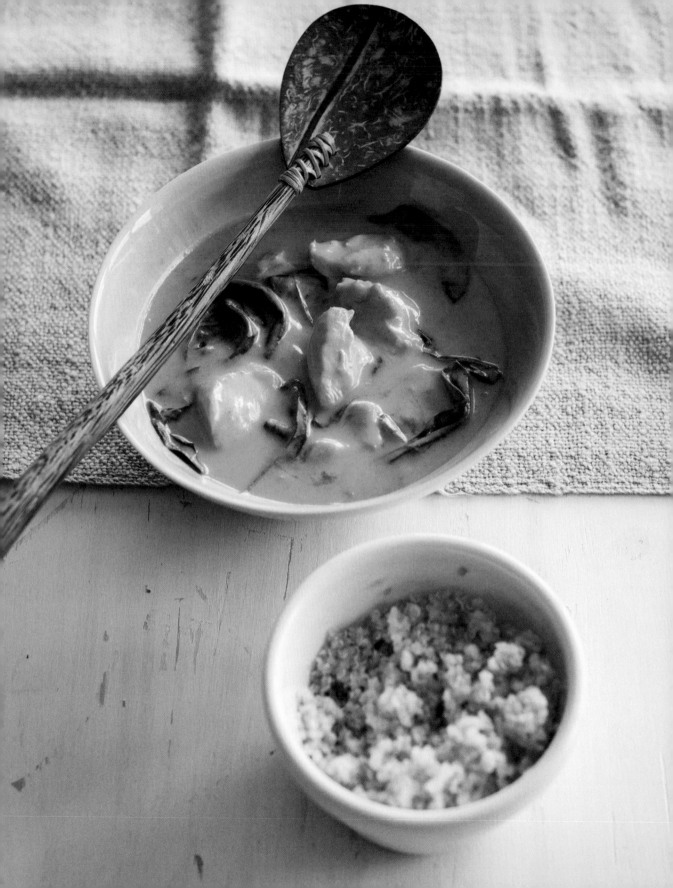

PCOS
Diet
for the
Newly
Diagnosed

Your All-In-One Guide to Eliminating PCOS
Symptoms with the Insulin Resistance Diet

TARA SPENCER

Foreword by Megan-Marie Stewart,
Founder of the PCOS Awareness Association

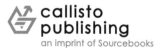
callisto
publishing
an imprint of Sourcebooks

Published by Callisto Publishing LLC C/O Sourcebooks LLC
P.O. Box 4410, Naperville, Illinois 60567-4410
(630) 961-3900
callistopublishing.com

Printed and bound in China
OGP 2

This book is dedicated to every woman
who has ever felt scared in her suffering.
You are not alone.

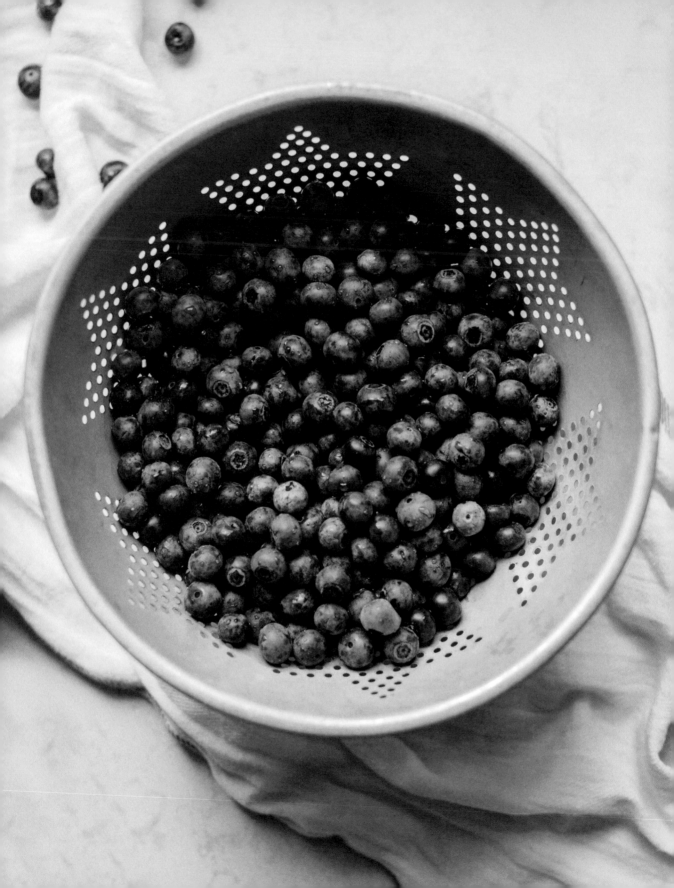

Contents

Foreword

I have struggled with Polycystic Ovarian Syndrome for most of my life and was finally diagnosed by my OB-GYN in 2000, when I was sixteen years old. At the time, I did not understand how serious the condition could be. It was not until 2005, when I was hospitalized due to cysts rupturing, that I finally understood the extent of my symptoms. The pain of the cysts rupturing was unbearable, and when I left the hospital, I decided that there had to be a better way to live.

I began doing research and discovered that I was not alone in this struggle. I decided to make it my mission to raise awareness of PCOS. I started selling handmade teal (the official color for PCOS) bracelets to friends and family, and before I knew it, I had people in England and Australia contacting me to request bracelets. Taking this as a sign of things to come, I took the funds and started the nonprofit organization, PCOS Awareness Association (PCOSAA). That was in 2012, and today we are the world's second largest nonprofit dedicated to Polycystic Ovarian Syndrome.

Over the last two years I have gone on a natural health path and have come off all the medications that used to keep my PCOS symptoms manageable (I do not suggest this without talking to a medical professional first). I eat healthier, exercise, and see a women's health acupuncturist. I have lost 50 lbs on this path, have gained my menstrual cycle back, and am healthier overall. While on this journey, I have noticed things that are missing or needed for women who want to control their PCOS naturally, and the *PCOS Diet for the Newly Diagnosed* fills the voids.

From weekly meal plans and grocery shopping lists to exercise routines and Daily Gratitude and Habit Tracker worksheets, this book is more than just delicious recipes.

We all have busy schedules, and due to my life situations, I fell off my health journey several months ago. This diet plan gave me my life again; my motivation is back, and I am ready to take control of my health once again. I began using the book soon after receiving it and I already feel refreshed and inspired to continue.

It is important to remember that nothing of worth comes for free or comes easily, but if you are willing to make a positive change and stick with it, results are inevitable. Having a positive support system is also key; I would never have been able to do what I have done (starting PCOSAA and taking control of my health) without the support of my family and friends. Women with PCOS often feel alone, unattractive and uninspired. Please know that you are not alone–you are beautiful and this book will inspire you.

Thank you, Tara, for taking the time to create a book that all women with PCOS can use as a helpful tool in taking control of their health.

MEGAN-MARIE STEWART
Founder of PCOS Awareness Association

ABOUT THE FOREWORD CONTRIBUTOR

Megan-Marie Stewart is the proud Founder and Executive Director of PCOS Awareness Association (www.pcosaa.org), the second largest nonprofit organization dedicated to Polycystic Ovarian Syndrome worldwide. Her vision and the mission of PCOS Awareness Association is to revolutionize PCOS awareness and fight on behalf of those who live with it.

Introduction

When I was first diagnosed with polycystic ovarian syndrome (PCOS), I felt shocked, scared, and worried about my future. I was in my early twenties and, like many women, fairly ignorant about the condition. After receiving my diagnosis, I assumed I would continue to be overweight, afflicted by acne, and unable to conceive for the rest of my life. I did not know that PCOS could be managed.

My doctor at the time was relatively unhelpful, merely suggesting I, once again, take birth control pills to normalize my hormones artificially. He reassured me that once I was ready to become pregnant I could use in vitro fertilization (IVF)— something most people know is not easy, cheap, or guaranteed to be successful.

I did research on my own, and learned that the underlying cause of my PCOS was insulin resistance. After years of an irregular menstrual cycle, painful cystic acne, and dreaded fat that clung to my middle, I was able to control my symptoms through diet and exercise.

All the pain and frustration surrounding my body throughout the preceding years finally made sense, but I was overwhelmed. I was trying everything, and the information available concerning PCOS seemed written for women aware and knowledgeable of their condition for some time; there were few sources to help the uninformed, newly diagnosed.

Although PCOS is common, affecting about 4 to 8 percent of women worldwide and as many as 25 percent in some populations (Traub 2011), I still felt extremely isolated; among other things, my friends did not have PCOS and could not relate to my suffering. I felt I had no one to turn to.

I quickly became an expert on PCOS. I spent years manipulating my diet and exercise routine, sculpting the perfect lifestyle to manage my symptoms naturally. I became more in tune with my body than ever before, and I increasingly appreciated the value of a healthy diet, a moderate exercise regime, and a stress-free life.

However, it was not all smooth sailing. In the early days following my diagnosis, I would often just curl up and cry: My job as a personal trainer is incredibly appearance-centric and it was disappointing to know

I'd never achieve the lean physique I longed for. When I was a newlywed, I was devastated at the possibility of never being able to conceive naturally. My PCOS diagnosis wasn't the end of the world, but at times it felt like it.

As a certified personal trainer and nutritionist, I'm in the business of helping people. I immediately wanted to help other women like me who felt lost and confused after their own diagnosis. I tried everything so others wouldn't have to. I became a PCOS specialist and have since worked with hundreds of women with the same condition.

I teach women to heal their bodies from the inside out as well as how to deal with insulin resistance and hormonal sensitivity. I stress the importance of loving your body, despite any physical ailments, and give hope that it is possible to restore fertility, abolish even the most severe acne, stop male-pattern hair growth, and lose unwanted pounds. I love what I do and find it very rewarding to watch women lead rich and full lives with PCOS.

In this book you will find a two-week meal plan (see pages 44 to 48) that contains easy-to-follow recipes to teach you how to overcome insulin resistance using your diet. In addition, chapter 2 contains a two-week, no-equipment exercise plan appropriate for beginners (see pages 31 to 37), which explains how to exercise enough to support proper hormonal functioning without overdoing it and causing further stress to your body. You may repeat and cycle the plans, spending two weeks learning to cook in a new way, and the following two weeks learning to add exercise to your lifestyle. I've also included Daily Gratitude and Habit Tracker worksheets (see pages 32 to 33) to help you track your progress (and feel proud of yourself!) as you learn to live a healthier lifestyle and record daily positive moments that can help stave off the stress of living with PCOS. After repeating these plans a few times, you will have all the tools and experience you need to maintain a healthy lifestyle. Although PCOS is not a curable condition, its symptoms can be managed to the point of being barely noticeable—and this book shows you how.

1

PCOS and
Metabolism
Repair

PCOS and insulin resistance are both common conditions, so there is a large amount of research available concerning both. I've recommended my favorite books, organizations, and websites in the Resources section (page 156). However, while there is a lot about PCOS and insulin resistance, there is little information about how the two conditions can be managed in tandem and dealing with the additional challenges that each brings.

Although PCOS can only be managed, not cured, its symptoms can be significantly improved by overcoming insulin resistance with your diet, and it is undeniably worth it to follow the dietary recommendations laid out in this book. Please remember: Always consult your health-care provider before embarking on any major changes to your lifestyle or diet.

PCOS—What You Need to Know

In basic terms, PCOS is a malfunction of the female reproductive system. It was once thought that a woman had PCOS if she was overweight with visible signs of excess androgens (male sex hormones), such as hair growth. The medical community now accepts that women with all kinds of body types and varying degrees of symptoms can have the condition.

PCOS is characterized by at least two of the following symptoms, usually confirmed with ultrasounds and/or hormonal blood tests:

- Blood sugar disorders (including insulin resistance)
- Cysts on the ovaries
- Difficulty conceiving
- Elevated levels of androgens
- Irregular or absent menstrual cycle

Despite what its name suggests, though, not every woman with PCOS has cysts on her ovaries, and not every woman with ovarian cysts has PCOS.

Androgens, often referred to as "male hormones," are present in both men and women. It is important to note, however, that a healthy woman typically produces only about 5 to 10 percent of the androgens produced by a man (Health Line 2015), and so is, therefore, more sensitive to their effects.

Testosterone, dihydrotestosterone, and androstenedione are the three principal androgens. When present in excessive amounts, they cause the common symptoms of PCOS such as acne, male-pattern hair growth (hirsutism), male-pattern hair loss (androgenic alopecia), depression, mood swings, sleep problems, excess weight gain, and difficulty losing weight.

Elevated androgen levels also interfere with the natural function of the four key hormones involved in the female menstrual cycle:

1. Follicle-stimulating hormone
2. Luteinizing hormone
3. Estrogen
4. Progesterone

In a normal cycle, an egg is produced and released by the ovaries into the fallopian tubes, where it becomes fertilized by a sperm and is carried to the uterus to develop as a fetus. If fertilization does not occur, the uterine lining is shed (menstruation). The entire process is highly complicated and depends on numerous hormones functioning together perfectly. It is easy to see how even one small glitch can throw the whole system out of whack.

If you have PCOS, the cycle just described is not as straightforward. Primarily because of the influence of androgens, the egg either does not develop, or it is not released during ovulation. If a woman's hormonal balance is not restored, androgens can have serious long-term consequences, such as the development of insulin resistance and diabetes, high cholesterol, high blood pressure, heart disease, infertility, depression, sleep apnea, metabolic

WHEN YOU DON'T LOVE
YOUR APPEARANCE–OR YOURSELF

PCOS doesn't just affect your menstrual cycle and fertility. It often displays outwardly in your appearance or weight, making it particularly challenging. You may find it difficult to treat yourself with kindness and your self-esteem may be low—and it is normal to feel this way.

While changing lifestyle choices to improve physical symptoms, it's also important to spend time cultivating a strong body image. Appreciate all the things your body can do, focus on the positive aspects of your appearance, and take time for yourself. Surround yourself with loving friends and family, avoid negative people and unrealistic media images, and speak to yourself in the same supportive manner you use with others. Everyone has physical hang-ups and unique journeys—do not compare yourself to others. I offer additional guidance in chapter 2, including Daily Gratitude and Habit Tracker worksheets (pages 32 to 33).

If you are dealing with androgenic symptoms, such as stubborn weight gain, acne, or hair growth, focus on positive actions you can control. Instead of hiding behind baggy clothes, wear flattering clothes that make you feel like a million dollars. Try topical hair removal creams, and apply makeup for a confidence boost. Exercising frequently will also make you feel better.

Know that, over time, you will see the positive effects of your lifestyle changes. You may notice your acne clearing, your dark body hair disappearing, or your weight dropping to a healthier level.

Patience and faith in yourself are key. Depending on the root cause of your PCOS, it may take longer for you to heal than others. Treat your body with love, kindness, and patience during the healing process.

syndrome, and ovarian and endometrial cancer. Women with PCOS who successfully become pregnant have a higher rate of miscarriage, gestational diabetes, and premature delivery.

Although it is difficult to establish the direct causes of PCOS, it is commonly linked to insulin resistance—often caused by a poor diet, excess weight, inflammation, stress, genetics, or a combination of these. As many as 70 percent of women with PCOS are insulin resistant (Traub 2011). Most people who are insulin resistant are overweight, as the two conditions beget each other.

At other times, the emergence of PCOS is linked to periods of significant physical or psychological stress. And while many women benefit from losing weight, underweight women—already in a stressed physical state—actually benefit from gaining weight.

In some women, the symptoms of PCOS appear soon after menstruation first begins, while others' PCOS is triggered years later. The cause of my PCOS is not necessarily the cause of your PCOS, so it is important to be patient and experiment with different factors until your body responds positively.

Despite being an incurable condition, there are ways to effectively manage PCOS and lead a normal, healthy life. By recognizing the symptoms early and proactively treating them, you will reduce your risk of diabetes, heart disease, infertility, and miscarriage. Regardless of which medical treatments your doctor recommends to manage your PCOS and insulin resistance, all women benefit from developing healthy dietary and exercise habits. Every affected woman will benefit from eliminating toxins, nourishing her body with natural foods, minimizing stress levels, and following an appropriate exercise routine. The following pages show you how to ensure your body is healthy, energetic, fertile, and pain-free.

A Healthy Diet and a Healthy Metabolism

When we eat a diet rich in natural, healthy foods, including slow-digesting, complex carbohydrates, our bodies can monitor our blood sugar levels, respond to the demands of the cells, and release insulin in precisely the right amounts. The healthier your diet is, the healthier your metabolism will be.

Metabolism can be affected by age, sex, genetics, height, and weight. It is increased through regular physical activity, and also by choosing types of exercise that increase lean muscle tissue, such as resistance training. You can read more about the ideal exercise regime for women with PCOS on pages 31 to 37. Obtaining an adequate amount of sleep and minimizing stress levels is also crucial to maintain a strong metabolism.

All overweight women with PCOS should try to lose weight. A 1992 study by Kiddy et al. showed that even a 5 to 7 percent reduction in body weight over a six-month period can lower insulin and androgen levels to restore ovulation and fertility in more than 75 percent of obese women with PCOS. Later studies have confirmed this (Norman et al. 2004).

Although it is important to lose weight when you are insulin resistant, remember not to reduce your calories too much, as that will slow your metabolism over time. Never drop below about 1,500 calories a day, as this is the minimum amount most women need for basic bodily functions.

The Connection between Insulin Resistance and PCOS

Insulin is a hormone that has an important connection to testosterone (also a hormone), which can intensify PCOS symptoms when present in elevated amounts. It is, therefore, imperative that once diagnosed with PCOS, you learn to keep your insulin levels normal.

Not every woman with PCOS has insulin resistance, or vice versa, but they are closely related. In a 2013 study by Stepto et al., 95 percent of overweight women with PCOS were insulin resistant, but so were 75 percent of lean women with PCOS. The high levels of insulin in the blood seen in insulin-resistant individuals increase testosterone production and can aggravate underlying PCOS symptoms. In turn, androgens also reduce the sensitivity of our body's receptors for insulin and create defects in the way our cells process or move glucose, worsening insulin resistance (Corbould 2008).

Some women may even be eating well and exercising regularly, but still find it difficult to lose weight. This is the influence of insulin resistance and, luckily, it can be managed.

The good news is that insulin resistance is a reversible (again, not curable) condition—losing weight, following a healthy diet, and exercising regularly all help the body respond better to insulin. This, in turn, reduces androgen production, which restores fertility, regulates the menstrual cycle, encourages weight loss, and abolishes the male-pattern symptoms of PCOS—all things I have successfully achieved, and you can, too.

Insulin and Metabolism

The primary hormone involved in regulating a person's metabolism is insulin. At mealtimes and at regular intervals throughout the day, your pancreas releases insulin to control the level of glucose in your blood. It is the hormone that allows your muscle, fat, and liver cells to take in nutrients, thereby lowering blood glucose levels. The cells either use the nutrients immediately for energy or store them for use at a later time. By working with your metabolism in this way, insulin is responsible for using digested food as energy, and so it fuels every process required to sustain life. In a healthy person, the process of metabolism functions to allow glucose and insulin levels to remain within a normal range.

Insulin resistance is a condition in which the body's cells do not respond properly to insulin and cannot absorb glucose from the bloodstream, meaning your body cannot convert food into energy. This can result when your body fails to produce enough insulin to meet demand, or when your cells build up a resistance to insulin.

So, although insulin is present in the bloodstream, it is not enough to trigger the cells to take in nutrients. The body starts demanding higher amounts of insulin to help glucose enter the cells, so the pancreas produces more and more insulin—but, eventually, the pancreatic cells will fail to keep up and will become damaged. Excess glucose will build up in the bloodstream and, even when it is finally absorbed by the cells, excess amounts of insulin will remain in the bloodstream, acting only to further confuse the pancreas. Any extra glucose has nowhere to go and is subsequently stored as fat, meaning one's body weight will gradually creep up over time. Eventually, this increasingly reduced sensitivity to the demands of insulin leads to diabetes, prediabetes, and other serious health problems.

According to the National Institute of Diabetes and Digestive and Kidney Diseases, the main causes of insulin resistance are being overweight, physical inactivity, ethnicity, hormonal problems, steroid use, sleep disorders, and smoking.

Excess belly fat produces hormones that can interfere with normal body function and contribute to chronic inflammation, both of which combine to cause insulin resistance. In what becomes a vicious cycle, insulin resistance slows your metabolism and makes it even more difficult for your body to break down and absorb highly refined, processed foods.

Physical activity encourages the body's muscle cells to burn their stored glucose for energy and refill their stores with glucose from the bloodstream (O'Neill 2013). This keeps blood glucose levels in check, and explains why it is so important for PCOS sufferers to follow the exercise recommendations in chapter 2 (pages 31 to 37).

Just as insulin resistance can result from being overweight due to physical inactivity and a nutrient-poor diet, it can also be caused by the opposite—low-calorie crash diets and excessive amounts of exercise. These create unwanted stress within the body, shut down normal hormonal production, and can trigger PCOS in young adult women.

Insulin resistance can be reversed and controlled by avoiding highly processed carbohydrates that have a high glycemic index, such as unrefined sugars and white flour products. These types of foods quickly increase blood glucose levels and require that greater amounts of insulin be secreted in response. By choosing foods lower on the glycemic index, such as whole-grain breads, brown rice, and nonstarchy vegetables, you can improve your insulin response. More details about the ideal diet for reversing insulin resistance follow (see page 39).

The medication metformin is often prescribed to treat type 2 diabetes and insulin resistance, but a study by the Diabetes Prevention Program (Bloomgarden 2009) showed that the drug's benefits were not as significant compared to a healthy diet and regular exercise. While it can sometimes be useful to rely on doctors and their prescriptions, we must never give up on our body's innate ability to heal itself.

The Purpose of Food

All food we eat is made up of three macronutrients, in varying degrees:

- Carbohydrate
- Protein
- Fat

During digestion, food is broken down into glucose, proteins, and micronutrients. As we know, glucose is used as the body's primary fuel source, while the other two digestive by-products are used for cellular metabolism, immune function, and cell replacement. These foods directly affect our metabolism and insulin response.

CARBOHYDRATE

The body's preferred source of energy is the carbohydrate, which is converted to glucose during digestion. Insulin-resistant women should avoid simple, quick-digesting types of carbohydrates such as chocolate, cookies, sweetened fruits, soda, and white-flour products, as they cause sudden peaks and dips in blood sugar levels. Instead, choose complex, slow-releasing forms of carbohydrates, such as beans, oatmeal, sweet potatoes, and brown-flour products. While carbohydrate intake should be controlled because it has a greater effect on insulin than the other macronutrients,

it should not be overly restricted, as that can cause greater problems when carbohydrates are reintroduced. As long as you select sources from the Foods to Enjoy list (see page 22), you can enjoy carbohydrates while also supporting a strong, healthy metabolism and working to reverse your insulin resistance.

PROTEIN

Protein allows the body to grow and repair its tissues, and is sometimes used as a source of energy. Protein has also been shown to speed metabolism (Paddon-Jones et al. 2008). The healthiest types of protein are lean meats and poultry, fish, eggs, and legumes.

FAT

The third and final macronutrient is fat. Most people assume fat is bad for their health, however this is not true for all fats. Saturated and trans fats, found in fatty animal products and processed foods, respectively, should be avoided. But consuming the right types of fat is essential to achieve optimal health. Monounsaturated and polyunsaturated fats—found in avocados, beef, nuts, olives, seeds, and oily fish—should be eaten in moderation, as they help process vitamins, protect internal organs, regulate body temperature, and repair body tissue.

The Insulin Resistance Diet for PCOS

One thing increasingly acknowledged is that food can act as medicine. Eating a diet composed of healthy, natural foods is the most important step you can take to treat your PCOS naturally.

Before turning to artificial medicines for help, women should address any controllable factors to improve their PCOS symptoms. The foods we eat send a direct message to our bodies about which hormones to produce and when. It is necessary to control our diets to reverse insulin resistance and balance androgen production. By starting with dietary modifications, you will teach your body that it does not need to rely on medicine to be healthy.

Interestingly, women who live in one of the few existing hunter-gather societies do not suffer from PCOS. PCOS appears to be something that has evolved as a result of the diet and lifestyle behaviors of Western society.

So, it makes sense that to manage PCOS symptoms we need to reconnect with a natural style of eating. This means eating nutrient-dense whole foods found in nature, such as lean meats, fresh fruits and vegetables, whole grains, nuts, and seeds, and simultaneously avoiding foods our ancestors would not recognize, such as processed and packaged snacks, soy products, and high-fructose corn syrup. The latter types of foods are filled with chemicals, confuse our body's natural insulin response, and cause hormonal disruptions.

Regardless of which specific hormone is triggering your PCOS–whether it is elevated testosterone, decreased DHEA-S, or increased estrogen or progesterone–nourishing your body with a healthy diet will improve your symptoms.

When on an insulin resistance diet for PCOS, follow these guidelines.

- **Avoid artificial sweeteners, dairy, gluten, soy, sugar, and trans fats.** Artificial sweeteners stimulate the release of insulin and wreak havoc on your hormonal system. Dairy and gluten can increase inflammation, erode gut health, and cause insulin resistance (Kresser 2010). Both dairy and soy are highly hormonal foods, and the presence of either in your system can interfere with natural hormone production. Sugar directly affects insulin production but also plays a significant role in obesity, which can result in developing insulin resistance. Trans fats also cause inflammation and metabolic distress, which gradually lead to fat storage and insulin resistance.

- **Consume a moderate amount of low glycemic index, high-fiber carbohydrates.** This includes brown rice, buckwheat, legumes, millet, non-starchy vegetables, quinoa, and all other foods on the Foods to Enjoy list (see page 22). These foods are released into your bloodstream slowly and will improve your insulin sensitivity.

- **Avoid refined, processed carbohydrates rich in toxins and chemicals.** This includes unrefined sugars and white flour, rice, and potatoes (but not sweet potatoes).

- **Carbohydrates should contribute 40 to 50 percent of your daily calories.** Women who are overweight can afford to eat slightly fewer carbohydrates, but all PCOS-afflicted women should eat at least 100 grams of carbohydrates per day to improve their insulin sensitivity. Protein calories should be equal to the calories from carbohydrates (40 to 50 percent), while fat calories should make up the balance (10 to 20 percent).

- **Eat small, frequent meals throughout the day.** Eat every three to four hours during the day to keep your blood sugar levels stable and prevent sudden, excessive demands for insulin caused by eating big meals. However, avoid continual snacking, as it interferes with the normal signaling and functioning of insulin and other hormones.

- **Eat a balance of lean protein, complex carbohydrates, and healthy fats at every meal.** Pay particular attention that you do not eat carbohydrates alone, such as a piece of fruit for a snack, because it will spike your blood sugar levels. Rather, combine carbohydrates with a protein and fat to slow digestion. For example, eat a piece of fruit with nut butter or cheese.

- **Eat organic protein when possible.** Organic and grass-fed lean meats, poultry, and eggs are free from excessive amounts of estrogen and antibiotics (which disrupt normal hormone production in humans), typically found in conventionally raised animal products.

- **Drink only water and noncaffeinated herbal teas.** Caffeine has been shown to increase insulin resistance by 15 percent (Biaggioni and Davis 2002), so avoid it. Sodas and juices are void of nutrients and filled with sugar, fructose, and glucose, while alcohol is a highly inflammatory toxin that you should also avoid.

- **Consider additional supplementation.** Along with a natural diet, certain supplements are linked to improved hormonal health and natural ovulation. These include calcium, chromium, coenzyme Q10, cod liver oil, DIM (diindolymethane), evening primrose oil, gymnema, iodine, magnesium, N-acetyl cysteine, selenium, taurine, vitamins B_6 and D, and zinc.

On the herbal front, vitex agnus castus, apple cider vinegar, cinnamon, fenugreek, flaxseed, licorice root, maca, milk thistle, saw palmetto, and spearmint tea are particularly beneficial for women with PCOS. I have responded well to agnus castus, DIM, and magnesium. Please see the Natural Fertility Info in the Resources section, page 156, for more information on supplements.

By following the preceding guidelines, you should naturally start to lose weight—assuming you need to—and improve your insulin sensitivity. Your caloric intake should fall naturally as you cut out all calorically dense processed foods. However, remember never to drop below about 1,500 calories a day, as that only creates further stress inside your already strained body.

While the principles of this diet are designed to help women overcome all general symptoms of PCOS, some recipes in this book are specifically targeted toward women trying to conceive, women who want to fight inflammation, or women trying to lose weight. They are labeled Fertility Boost, Inflammation Fighter, and Lower Calorie. Some recipes also include tips with the same names to help you identify and address your specific needs.

By adhering to the foods recommended in the following table, you will soon overcome your insulin resistance and, in turn, your PCOS.

Foods to Enjoy and Foods to Avoid

FOODS TO ENJOY

- Dairy alternatives (almond milk, coconut milk, and hazelnut milk)
- Dark chocolate
- Eggs
- Fish (cod, halibut, herring, salmon, sardines)
- Garlic
- Lean meats (beef, chicken, lamb, pork, turkey)
- Legumes (black beans, chickpeas, lentils, soybeans)
- Low glycemic index fruits (apples, berries, cherries, peaches, pears, plums, rhubarb)
- Low glycemic index vegetables (asparagus, broccoli, Brussels sprouts, cabbage, kale, spinach)
- Medium glycemic index fruits (cantaloupes, grapes, kiwi)
- Nuts and seeds (almonds, flaxseed, macadamia nuts, pumpkin seeds, walnuts)
- Oils (coconut oil, extra-virgin olive oil, flaxseed oil)
- Whole grains (amaranth, buckwheat, millet, quinoa, teff)

FOODS TO AVOID

- Alcohol
- All foods containing high-fructose corn syrup (breakfast cereals, juices, ketchup, salad dressings, sodas)
- All foods containing hydrogenated oils (cakes, candy, chips, doughnuts)
- All foods containing white sugar and white flour (bagels, breads, cereals, pasta, pastries)
- Artificial sweeteners (acesulfame, aspartame, saccharin, sorbitol)
- Dairy, most
- Fish containing mercury (swordfish, tuna, tilefish)
- High glycemic index vegetables (corn, parsnips, white potatoes, rutabagas, turnips)
- Processed fruit juices
- Processed oils (canola, corn, peanut, safflower, sunflower)
- Red meat (unless organic or grass fed) and organ meats

NOW THAT YOU KNOW, WHAT'S NEXT?

When I received my PCOS diagnosis, I was shocked, scared, and nervous. I wish someone had been by my side to reassure me that everything would be okay, and tell me I was not doomed to a lifetime of being overweight, acne-ridden, and infertile. Here are some things I wish I had known at that time that may help you.

Initially, you must track your PCOS symptoms and food intake:

To determine what aggravates your symptoms, it is crucial to keep a record of your menstrual cycle and other PCOS-related symptoms, such as acne, hair growth, and changes in body weight. Also, take note of the food you eat every day and the exercise you do. Soon you will see the connection between dietary and lifestyle behaviors and your PCOS.

PCOS does not make you infertile:

It is possible to conceive naturally—or, at least, with the help of fertility drugs.

Tackling PCOS requires lifestyle changes and patience. To manage symptoms, you must avoid negative behaviors that may aggravate PCOS, such as smoking, not sleeping enough, and eating too much junk food. Learning to nurture your body takes time, but produces worthwhile results.

You are not alone:

PCOS is a common condition, and it is very easy to connect with others online (my favorite forums are listed in the Resources section, page 156).

There are alternative solutions:

In addition to your medical doctor, consider an endocrinologist or alternative medicine practitioner, such as an acupuncturist. To deal with the emotional strain of PCOS, it may be helpful to consult a therapist.

Setting Reasonable Expectations

Some women respond positively and immediately after beginning the plan detailed in this book, while others may respond negatively. It depends on how healthy your diet is to begin with.

If you do experience negative side effects after beginning this diet, any negative side effects are usually moderate and short-lived. Remind yourself of the long-term benefits. Overcoming a few cravings, headaches, and reduced energy levels for the first few days are worth it to regain a regular menstrual cycle, improve your fertility and insulin sensitivity, and experience weight loss over time—and feel better overall.

Short-Term Changes

If you have been consuming a standard American diet, typically containing inflammatory and toxic foods, your body will initially go into shock when starting a healthier diet, and you may experience some negative symptoms. The good news is these symptoms only last a few days or, at most, a couple of weeks before you start reaping the long-term benefits of this diet.

CRAVINGS AND HEADACHES

Processed foods contain addictive properties, so when you first remove these foods from your diet, you will likely experience strong cravings and headaches. These will stop once their toxins are completely removed from

your bloodstream, and you will eventually crave the healthier fresh fruits and vegetables you are introducing instead.

DIPS IN ENERGY LEVELS

High-calorie processed foods provide quick bursts of energy. By eliminating these foods, you may initially feel more lethargic. However, others might experience increased energy once they start fueling their bodies with healthier, more nutritious foods. In the end, everyone will benefit from higher energy levels and improved sleep.

WEIGHT LOSS

Many women lose weight almost immediately after beginning this diet, particularly if they simultaneously follow the exercise plan in chapter 2 (pages 31 to 37). You will naturally be eating fewer calories than before, as well as fewer foods that encourage fat storage in insulin-resistant individuals.

The exact rate of weight loss will depend on the individual, but it should feel natural and almost effortless. And, as your insulin sensitivity continues to improve, you will continue to lose weight. As we know, even mild weight loss can significantly improve PCOS symptoms, so this is a very important benefit.

Long-Term Changes

Now that we have the negative short-term effects out of the way, let's focus on the positive aspects of the diet. Please be patient—it can take six months before you see any major improvements in your PCOS symptoms. Your body is doing the best it can to heal, but it can't rush the process. So be kind to yourself and remember you're giving yourself the gift of a healthier diet and lifestyle—and that's awesome.

FEWER CYSTS

If you have cysts on your ovaries, they will reduce in number once your hormonal health improves. This, in turn, reduces any associated abdominal pain.

HEIGHTENED INSULIN SENSITIVITY

This diet will improve your insulin resistance and, in turn, reduce androgen production.

FEWER MALE-PATTERN SYMPTOMS

Once you improve your insulin sensitivity and thereby reduce your androgen production, you will experience fewer male-associated PCOS symptoms, such as acne, hair growth, and baldness.

IMPROVED DIGESTION

Dairy, gluten, and sugar negatively affect our digestive systems. Once you remove these foods from your diet, you will experience less bloating, constipation, and diarrhea as well as more regular bowel movements.

IMPROVED MOODS

Women with PCOS are commonly affected by mood swings, which are worsened by the spikes and drops in blood sugar caused by high-carbohydrate and high-fat foods. By

PRACTICAL LIFESTYLE TIP

Incorporate small bursts of activity into your daily routine. Set hourly timers on your phone to take a five-minute walk, perform 20 jumping jacks, or climb a few flights of stairs.

replacing these foods with slow-releasing options, you will feel less irritable and your concentration levels will improve.

LOWER BLOOD PRESSURE AND INFLAMMATION

When you eat a healthy diet low in sugar, saturated fat, and trans fat, your blood pressure will fall. This means you are at reduced risk of heart attack, heart disease, stroke, and other diseases (American Heart Association 2016). Avoiding highly inflammatory foods, such as dairy, gluten, and soy, also improves your immunity.

RESTORED FERTILITY

Following this diet will improve your fertility, as it will improve the signaling between your pituitary gland and your ovaries. This will increase your chances of ovulating and conceiving naturally, better prepare your uterus for implantation, and reduce your risk of miscarriage as well as insulin resistance developing into diabetes (Natural Fertility Info 2016).

2

Living Well to Eat Well

Although ensuring that your diet is primarily composed of healthy, nutrient-dense foods is the most important natural method to overcoming insulin resistance, there are other lifestyle factors you must evaluate and modify to accelerate your journey to optimal health and vitality. These include:

- Achieving adequate rest and sleep

- Taking time to destress through pleasurable activities

- Exercising regularly to increase insulin sensitivity

Developing a healthier emotional relationship with your body is extremely important during this stage, so this chapter also covers mindful eating (see page 39) and how to manage your relationships with others successfully (see page 38). Each woman's PCOS is triggered for a different reason, so each woman has her own journey of self-discovery and experimentation ahead. Provided you follow the guidelines here, you will see progress day by day.

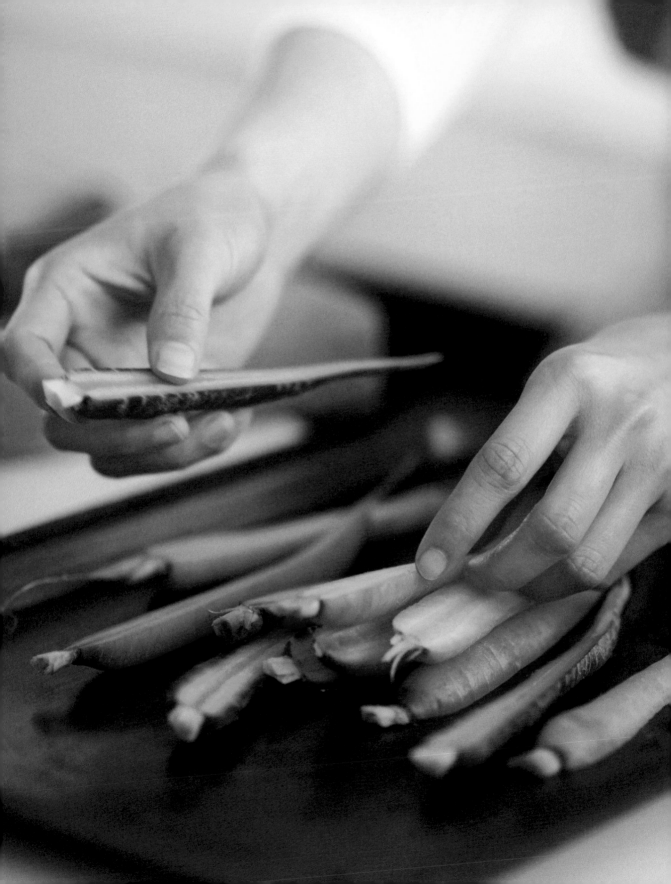

The Importance of a Healthy Lifestyle

Physical activity has a particularly positive effect on reversing insulin resistance, and this is covered in more detail later in this chapter (pages 31 to 37). It is also important to ensure you are well rested and happy, as mood and stress levels strongly influence insulin, cortisol, and androgen production (Ranabir and Reetu 2011). It is all the more important for women trying to conceive to address these factors to create an optimal environment for fertilization.

Rest and Sleep

For some with a predisposition, PCOS can be triggered by poor sleep patterns. Lack of sleep causes insulin resistance and increases cortisol production. Cortisol is a hormone released in response to stress and, in normal amounts, it controls blood sugar levels, regulates metabolism, reduces inflammation, and maintains blood pressure. But in high amounts, cortisol sends mixed signals to the pituitary gland—which is responsible for hormone production—and it can also cause weight gain, high blood pressure, and mood swings.

As hormone production and healing peak during sleep, ensuring you have between seven and nine hours of shut-eye each night is essential to maintain proper metabolism and insulin response. Numerous studies have shown (including Knutson 2007 and Kondracki 2012) that

poor sleep habits contribute to an increased appetite—which is also linked to making unwise food decisions—and an increased rate of fat storage.

To improve your sleep hygiene and general rest habits, try the following tips.

- **Sleep for seven to nine hours a night, in a completely dark, quiet, and cool room.** Block all outside light with heavy curtains, blackout shades, or a sleep mask and muffle outside noise with earplugs or a sound machine. Keep your bedroom cool, but not too cool—the ideal temperature is around 65 degrees. Invest in a good-quality mattress and pillow.

- **Sleep and wake up at the same time every day.** Maintaining a regular sleep-wake cycle, or circadian rhythm, optimizes sleep quality and promotes streamlined hormonal production. Limit daytime naps to no more than 20 to 30 minutes—and only if absolutely necessary—and do not sleep in on weekends.

- **Eat a small, protein-rich snack about one hour before bed.** You should not go to bed hungry, but you should also not be overly full, as both cause discomfort and interfere with sleep.

- **Switch off electronics at least one hour before bed.** Mobile phones, tablets, computers, televisions, and other electronics emit bright lights that interfere with your body's natural sleep signals and, in turn, prevent you from falling into a deep sleep. If you must use a computer in the evening, install light-dimming software.

- **Exercise regularly.** Physical activity increases energy levels throughout the day and makes it easier to fall asleep at night. That said, avoid exercising within three hours of bedtime.

- **Avoid caffeine and other stimulants for six to eight hours before bed.** Do not consume coffee, tea, chocolate, energy drinks, or other stimulants such as nicotine and alcohol before you lie down.

- **Reserve your bed for sleep only.** Do not watch television or bring your laptop into your bed, as doing so will keep your mind active. Instead, keep a notepad on your bedside table to write down any pressing thoughts or worries, and deal with them in the morning.

- **In addition to good sleep behaviors, spend 30 to 60 minutes each day unwinding from the stresses of daily life.** A good time to do this is right before you go to sleep each night. Read, listen to music, meditate, or spend quality time with a loved one.

Pleasure and Joy

When a woman is stressed by environmental factors, the production of most of her hormones will fall—except the production of DHEA-S, which will increase in response to elevated cortisol. DHEA-S acts as an androgen and aggravates the symptoms of PCOS.

Stress has many forms—work, relationships, money-related concerns. Sometimes, too, it takes the form of years of undereating and overexercising, which will also increase cortisol levels, reduce pituitary activity, boost insulin production, increase inflammation, and elevate your risk of illness and chronic disease.

Stress affects both over- and underweight women with PCOS. In some cases, it pushes hormone production into overdrive; in other cases, it causes cessation. In a 1999 study by Ferin, monkeys placed within greater stressed environments suffered irregular periods and impaired fertility, despite being fed the same diet as the nonstressed group. When stressed, your body thinks it is not an ideal time for reproduction, so it shuts down normal functioning, which means it is imperative to manage your stress levels. The following advice should help:

- **Engage in at least one stress-relieving activity per day.** Meditation, yoga, reading, relaxing in a warm bath, and spending time with family and friends all relieve some symptoms of depression, anxiety, and stress. Doing something you enjoy should not be considered a luxury but rather an essential part of your daily life. Exercise can also help immensely with stress relief.

- **Reduce, or completely eliminate, all stress-causing activities.** This includes undereating, fasting, overexercising, smoking, and not getting enough sleep.
- **Use resources for guidance.** You can download mobile applications, audio recordings on Amazon, and instructional videos on YouTube to guide you through meditation or yoga. You can also find relaxation-focused groups on Meetup.com.
- **Practice self-compassion.** Express sympathy toward your own failures, inadequacies, and sufferings. Treat yourself with the same kindness you treat your loved ones.

Your Two-Week Exercise Plan

All types of physical activity encourage your body to use its stored glucose and, therefore, promote a proper hormonal balance and functioning metabolism. The effect is almost immediate. Adams's 2013 study demonstrated that a single bout of moderate-intensity exercise can increase glucose uptake and insulin sensitivity for between 24 and 72 hours after exercise.

Regular exercise also helps alleviate depression and anxiety commonly found in women with PCOS. It also helps overweight women lose weight, which we know is an important part of reversing insulin resistance and managing PCOS.

Another study (Hutchinson et al. 2011) showed that positive changes occur from exercise, even without weight loss. Women who exercised for three hours per week over a 12-week period improved their insulin sensitivity and lost visceral fat, despite not losing weight. The beneficial impact of exercise on insulin resistance is magnified if combined with a reduction in body weight and/or body fat.

For overweight women, normal amounts of exercise can improve fertility; however, extreme exercise patterns can cause the cessation of menstruation (amenorrhea) and infertility (Collins and Rossi 2015). Interestingly, a 2009 study by Gudmundsdottir, Flanders, and Augestad found that women who were active daily were 3.2 times more likely to have fertility problems than inactive women. But women who exercised a moderate amount (between 16 and 60 minutes per day) had a lower risk of infertility compared to women who exercised 15 or fewer minutes per day.

Therefore, the sweet spot appears to be exercising for about 30 minutes at least five days per week, but not to the point of exhaustion.

If you need motivation to kick-start your exercise regime, consider the following tips:

- **Keep in mind the benefits of both resistance training and aerobic exercise.** The former will build metabolically active muscle tissue, while the latter increases insulin sensitivity and reduces blood sugar levels.

DAILY GRATITUDE

Use this daily gratitude tracker to record moments for which you're thankful. Be specific, and try to notice something different every day so that your mind stays alert for new reasons to be grateful.

Use the habit tracker on page 33 to mark the days when you succeed in maintaining healthy habits. Keep the list of habits reasonable and realistic, and track them for at least 30 days before moving on to new habits.

M	*I am thankful for the 10-minute walk I was able to enjoy on my lunch break.*
T	
W	
TH	
F	
S	
SU	
M	
T	
W	
TH	
F	
S	
SU	

HABIT TRACKER

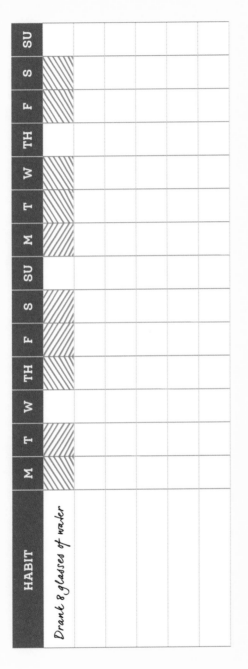

HABIT	M	T	W	TH	F	S	SU	M	T	W	TH	F	S	SU
Drank 8 glasses of water														

HABIT	M	T	W	TH	F	S	SU	M	T	W	TH	F	S	SU

- **Find a form of exercise you enjoy and do not view it as punishment.** While the following workout plan is ideal for PCOS sufferers, it is not compulsory. If you are more likely to stick to a regular yoga class, daily nature hike, or morning dip in the pool, choose that activity.

- **Treat your workouts as any other important appointment.** Schedule your workouts and honor your gym dates. If time is limited, split your workouts into short bursts of activity throughout the day—three 10-minute workouts during the day have the same positive effect as one 30-minute session.

The following exercise plan is perfect for beginners, as it does not require a gym membership or any expensive equipment. If you're brand new to some of these exercises (or it's been many years since you last learned to do them), then please proceed with caution and try them very slowly at first. It may help to ask a fitness-savvy friend or a personal trainer to provide some initial guidance since they will be able to watch your form as you move through the exercises. In general, you want to keep your back straight and your shoulders relaxed as you move.

The website exrx.net offers free descriptions and videos of the following exercises. Be sure not to push yourself too hard from the get-go; repeating the weekly plan twice will be a good start to your program.

Monday: 30-Minute Resistance Workout

Rest for 60 seconds between each exercise set. Complete all sets of one exercise before moving on to the next exercise.

SQUATS

4 x 12 repetitions

1. Stand with your feet hip-width apart and extend your arms straight out in front of you.
2. Push your hips back and squat down until your thighs are parallel with the ground.
3. Fully straighten your legs and squeeze your glutes when back in the standing position.
4. Repeat.

PUSH-UPS

4 x as many repetitions as possible
(Note: If regular push-ups on your toes are too difficult, do them standing with your hands placed against a wall or on an elevated surface.)

1. Place your hands shoulder-width apart on the floor, with your legs extended behind you, toes tucked under.
2. Lower your chest to one inch above the ground and push yourself back up.
3. Repeat.

LUNGES

4 x 10 repetitions (per side)

1. Stand with your feet together. With one foot, take a big step forward.

2. Lower your back knee to one inch above the ground, and then use your extended front leg to push back to a standing position.

3. Repeat all repetitions on one side before switching to the other side.

BURPEES

4 x 10 repetitions

(Note: For a lower-impact version, perform the exercise without jumping.)

1. Stand with your feet shoulder-width apart.

2. Push your hips back and squat to the floor.

3. Jump into a push-up position.

4. Reverse the motion to return to standing.

5. Repeat.

BICYCLE CRUNCHES

4 x 20 repetitions

1. Lie on your back with your hands behind your head; feet on the floor, knees bent.

2. Bring your right knee up, simultaneously lifting your upper back and shoulders off the floor, to meet your left elbow, keeping your left leg straight (not touching the floor).

3. Repeat, alternating sides.

Tuesday: 30-Minute Aerobic Workout

Take a brisk walk, jog, swim, or participate in a fitness class.

Wednesday: 30-Minute Resistance Workout

Rest for 60 seconds between each exercise set. Complete all sets of one exercise before moving on to the next exercise.

JUMPING JACKS

4 x 30 seconds

1. Stand with your feet together, hands by your sides.

2. Jump your feet out to the side while raising and clapping your hands overhead.

3. Jump your feet back together and bring your hands down.

4. Repeat.

GLUTE BRIDGES

4 x 20 repetitions

1. Lie on your back with your knees bent, feet on the floor.

2. Raise your hips, squeeze your glutes hard, and lower your hips to the floor.

3. Repeat.

STEP-UPS

4 x 10 repetitions (per side)

1. Stand facing a step or chair.
2. Place one foot on the surface and stand up, lifting your second leg.
3. Place your second foot back on the floor.
4. Repeat all repetitions on one side before switching to the other side.

SIDE LUNGES

4 x 10 repetitions (per side)

1. Standing with your feet together, toes pointed forward, take a big step out to the side with your right foot.
2. Keeping your back straight, lean into the lunge like you would a squat, until your right leg reaches a 90-degree angle and your left is straight. Push back and return to the starting position.
3. Repeat all repetitions on one side before switching to the other side.

TRICEPS DIPS

4 x as many repetitions as possible

1. Place your hands on the front edge of a chair or a step (as if you were going to sit on the chair), and walk your feet forward with either bent or straight legs.
2. Lower your body from the surface until your upper arms are parallel to the ground.
3. Push yourself back up.
4. Repeat.

DONKEY KICKS

4 x 10 repetitions (per side)

1. Get on your hands and knees, with your wrists under your shoulders and your knees under your hips.
2. Lift one leg parallel to the floor, with your knee bent and foot flexed.
3. Return to the starting position.
4. Repeat all repetitions on one side before switching to the other.

Thursday: 30-Minute Aerobic Workout

Take a brisk walk, a jog, swim, or participate in a fitness class.

Friday: 30-Minute Resistance Workout

For this workout, you will perform the exercises as a circuit–doing one set of each exercise with little rest in between. Once you complete one set of all seven exercises, rest for two minutes before completing the circuit an additional three times.

PRISONER SQUATS

12 repetitions

1. Follow the sequence for Squats (see page 34), but place your hands on either side of your head while doing the exercise.
2. Repeat.

JUMP LUNGES

20 repetitions (Note: For a lower-impact option, do 20 regular Lunges; see page 35).

1. Assume a lunge position (see page 35) with bent knees.
2. Jump straight up to switch legs.
3. Repeat.

HIGH KNEES

30 seconds

Run in place, raising your knees above hip level while pumping your arms.

MOUNTAIN CLIMBERS

30 seconds

1. In a Push-Up position (see page 34), bring one knee up toward your chest.
2. Change legs either by jumping or lightly stepping your feet forward and backward as quickly as possible.
3. Repeat for 30 seconds.

POP SQUATS

20 repetitions (Note: For a lower-impact option, do 20 regular Squats; see page 34).

1. Start standing with your feet together, knees slightly bent.
2. Jump up and land in a squat position with your thighs parallel to the floor.
3. Drive upward to jump again and land with your feet together.
4. Repeat.

WALL SIT

30 seconds

1. Standing next to a wall, slide your back down the wall until your thighs are parallel to the ground.
2. Keep your knees over your ankles and hold the position for 30 seconds.

PLANK

30 seconds

1. Assume a Push-Up position (see page 34).
2. Brace your core and hold your body in a straight line for 30 seconds.

Saturday: 30-Minute Aerobic Workout

Take a brisk walk, a jog, swim, or participate in a fitness class.

Sunday

Take a walk, do yoga, or rest.

Relationship Advice for Women with PCOS

Given the impact of PCOS on our physical and emotional health and appearance, it is natural for its effects to spill over into other parts of our lives, including our relationships. You may find yourself short-tempered with lovers, family members, or friends and you may struggle to start new relationships.

Trying to Conceive

If you received your PCOS diagnosis when you were trying to conceive, it may place a strain on your relationship. It is important to note that, although it may take time and patience to become pregnant, it is possible. Communicate your fears and concerns with your partner to protect your relationship. Never assume you know what your partner is thinking or feeling.

You may need to see a fertility specialist if your cycle is very irregular or absent, or if your periods are very heavy. Your specialist may prescribe fertility medications to induce egg development and ovulation, or IVF may be recommended. However, it is possible to have a healthy pregnancy and birth without these. Take your partner to appointments, address any side effects as a team, and grieve and celebrate together. Also, prioritize your relationship—schedule specific times when you are not allowed to discuss fertility struggles or PCOS.

It may be difficult for couples to maintain a healthy sex life during this recovery time—the woman may feel down about herself and sex can begin to feel like a chore. So, again, it is important to communicate openly about your feelings.

For women working through fertility issues, I recommend visiting Resolve and the Infertility Network websites (see Resources, page 156). You might also consider seeing a couples therapist. Remember, even if you feel alone, PCOS is the leading cause of infertility in the Western world, and one in eight couples of childbearing age has trouble conceiving or sustaining a pregnancy (Resolve 2015).

It can be helpful for your partner to understand the science behind PCOS—and reading this book can be a start. Always remember that PCOS can initially seem worse than it is, when your symptoms are not yet under control.

Single and Dating

If you are single and feeling self-conscious about the appearance-related burdens of PCOS, it may help to wait a month or two after starting this diet, to control some of your symptoms and regain some confidence, before throwing yourself back into the dating pool.

Friends and Family

Enlist support. Explain to your friends and family that you need to make a few dietary and lifestyle changes to help manage your condition. Tell them it would help enormously if they could jump on board with the changes, too—they may also enjoy a new, active lifestyle and a delicious new style of eating!

Stay in the moment and focus on one day at a time. With loved ones by your side, you should be able to conquer your PCOS in no time–and you may come out the other side with even stronger relationships.

Intuitive Eating and Mindfulness

It is unrealistic to expect to overcome insulin resistance within two weeks of beginning this plan. Rather, your short-term goal should be to establish a healthy new way of eating and an active and reduced-stress life, with a long-term goal to overcome insulin resistance.

The *PCOS Diet for the Newly Diagnosed* teaches you how to eat a healthy diet, but over time your goal should be to move away from a rigid meal plan. Instead, eat intuitively. This means developing a healthy relationship with your food, mind, and body by choosing to eat the right foods in the right quantities. This not only tunes you into your body's natural hunger and satiety signals, but is also the best means of nurturing your health and hormones as you naturally gravitate toward foods than make you feel good–inside and out. Intuitive eating moves us away from the idea of a strict diet and food avoidance and toward the proper understanding of food and why our bodies crave and thrive off different foods.

Follow these instructions for intuitive eating:

- **Listen to your natural hunger signals to determine when it is time to eat.** Do not eat according to the clock or another person's schedule. Do not get trapped by fad diets or restrictive meal plans–they do not work in the long run. Remember, we were born with the tools to eat intuitively, but they have become clouded by the diet industry and rigid food rules.

- **Be mindful when you eat.** Eat slowly, focus on the food in front of you, and put your utensils down between each bite. Eat until you feel comfortably full. Do not watch TV or surf the Internet while you eat.

- **Avoid emotional eating.** Do not turn to food in times of stress, depression, anxiety, or boredom. While food may provide short-term comfort, it will never solve the underlying problem and may, in fact, make you feel worse. To determine whether you are truly hungry, drink a glass of water and wait 15 minutes while doing something unrelated to food. Now how do you feel? Remind yourself of the true purpose of food and find alternative measures to improve your mood.

- **Pay attention to how your body reacts to certain foods.** In addition to following the advice for food choices (see Foods to Enjoy and Foods to Avoid, page 22), you should also keep a food journal to document how you feel, physically and emotionally, after eating. Over time, you should find you feel healthiest and most vibrant after consuming nutritious whole foods. You should naturally begin avoiding toxic foods (containing gluten, dairy, soy, and sugar), as they leave you feeling subpar and lacking energy. Do not place any foods off-limits, as you will likely only want to eat them more, but focus on the foods that make you feel great.

Before you can attempt intuitive eating, however, you must first cement your new healthy habits by following the two-week meal plan. All recipes contained within it are designed to be quick, convenient, and simple. Many can be prepared in just 30 minutes or less, or require a limited number of main ingredients. Most recipes generate leftovers, and all use ingredients that are wholesome, easy to find, and affordable. Above all, the recipes are delicious and were created to help you feel excited about your healthy new lifestyle!

Troubleshooting Tips

If you are willing to make some simple dietary changes and begin a straightforward exercise program, you can control your insulin resistance and, in turn, gain control over your PCOS symptoms. Although issues may arise, there is really no excuse not to take charge of your health and make the most of the factors within your control.

Here are 10 common problems (with helpful suggestions) you might face when beginning the meal plan in the *PCOS Diet for the Newly Diagnosed*.

1. **Lack of motivation:** It can feel overwhelming to think about overhauling your entire diet and lifestyle. Remind yourself why it is important to your health and wellness to nourish your body with a natural, whole-foods diet. Rather than changing your entire diet overnight and throwing yourself into an intense new exercise regimen, start with small, manageable steps. Spend one week simply learning about PCOS and mentally preparing for a change. Use the second week to review the meal plans and recipes, gauging how much time you will need to shop and cook, and to make room in your schedule. Once you begin using the meal plans, focus only on that for two weeks, taking breaks with pleasurable, self-compassionate activities whenever you feel tired or stressed. Once you feel comfortable with the healthier eating habits, begin integrating the two-week exercise plan into your lifestyle. By building these into your daily life, you can now make informed choices about what is best for your health. You have all the tools to benefit from the advice in this book.

2. **Lack of time:** You may feel you do not have time to eat healthy or exercise. About half the recipes in this book take only 15 to 30 minutes–start to finish–to prepare, which is about as long as it takes to grab takeout; other recipes require only a few ingredients and are easy to prepare. In some cases, you can even use already prepared ingredients and make food in bulk amounts. Instead of slumping in front of the TV after work, fit in a short workout first. If you are truly in a time crunch, do three 10-minute workouts each day instead of one longer session. Your health is something you must prioritize; you cannot afford not to make time for it.

3. **Lack of money:** It is not expensive to eat healthy. By avoiding takeout, restaurant meals, and nutritionally void junk food, you may actually save money. The exercise plan in this book does not require any special equipment or a gym membership. Over the long term, your investments in your health will pay for themselves in reduced medical bills.

4. **Information overload:** There is a lot of information out there about the best diet to follow for optimal health and weight loss. You may be confused about which foods are the healthiest, and which are off limits. Thankfully (and helpfully), all you need to know is contained within this book. Provided you follow its advice, you will see an improvement in your PCOS symptoms.

5. **Emotional eating and cravings:** The longer you stick with the principles of this diet, the fewer cravings you will experience. When you are tempted to eat for emotional reasons, remind yourself that doing so will simply distract you and does not address the real issue. Create a list of non-food-related activities that provide you pleasure, and turn to it whenever a craving hits. Remind yourself that a fleeting craving is not worth sacrificing all your hard work. Consider seeing a therapist if your food issues border on disordered eating behavior.

6. **Dislike of healthy foods:** We are often convinced that healthy foods are flavorless and unappealing compared to sweets and high-fat foods. This is because sugary, fatty, and salty foods frequently dull our taste buds over time, eventually making us need more to achieve the same level of satisfaction. Fortunately, it's also true that if you eat less of a particular food, you need less of it to feel satisfied. To change your food preferences, taper off the junk food little by little, and boost the sensual experience of eating healthy foods by appreciating smells and textures, savoring flavors, and appreciating the experience around eating. Play soft music and invite a friend over for good conversation. You can also mix new foods with some of your favorite foods so that, over time, your brain forms a positive association between both tastes. Within a few weeks,

you will notice your palate is more sensitive, and the flavors of healthy foods will be less dull or unappealing.

7. **Dislike of exercise:** It is important to find a form of exercise you enjoy to increase your likelihood of sticking with it. Because getting into "exercise mode" is half the battle of starting an exercise routine, minimize any potential obstacles that could slow you down. Keep your exercise clothes, hair tie, sneakers, and socks by the door and ready to go. Leave a corner of your home cleared so you can begin exercising right away, without having to move furniture or set up equipment. Mix in a highly enjoyable activity with your exercise workouts, such as watching a TV show or listening to a podcast. Even better, reserve your favorite, most addictive TV show for exercise times only, so you will start to look forward to your workouts; no exercise workout, no *Game of Thrones*. Finally, end your workouts with a relaxing cooldown in which you savor the satisfaction of getting in a good workout and congratulate yourself for moving your body.

8. **Criticism from friends and family:** Your loved ones may not understand why this diet is so important to your health, and they may attempt to lead you astray, tempting you with toxic, processed foods. Stress the importance of their support. Involve your family in the cooking process, and eat with friends who make you feel comfortable—rather than ashamed—about your food choices.

9. **Social temptations:** There will be times when available food choices do not fall in line with the principles of the *PCOS Diet for the Newly Diagnosed*. It is not reasonable (or realistic) to expect you will never indulge in sugar, dairy, or gluten again, but you must know when to do so and how to moderate your intake. Acknowledge that an occasional slip-up can happen and does not make you a failure, and make these occasions a rarity. It is also possible to attend parties and eat in restaurants without veering from the plan—stick to grilled meat or fish with fresh vegetables.

10. **Not enjoying water:** Instead of drinking plain water all the time (which grows tiring for anyone!) infuse it with cucumber, ginger, lemon, lime, mint, or orange. While you should limit caffeine consumption, you may drink green and herbal teas to your heart's content.

Pantry Staples

The key to following a healthy diet is stocking your kitchen with ingredients that are wholesome and nutritious, and used often in recipes in this book. You will be less likely to stray from your culinary plan if you always have the products you need at your fingertips. When planning your meals for the week, consult the shopping lists first, and when given a choice, add that item to your pantry and check off the items you already have.

- Almond butter, natural
- Arrowroot powder
- Baking powder
- Baking soda
- Beans (black, white, chickpeas, or lentils)
- Black pepper, freshly ground
- Broth, sodium-free (vegetable, chicken, or beef)
- Chia seeds
- Cinnamon, ground
- Coconut aminos
- Cooking spray, olive oil
- Flour, almond
- Flour, coconut
- Honey, raw
- Nuts (almonds, cashews, hazelnuts, pecans, pistachios, or walnuts)
- Oats, rolled
- Oil, extra-virgin olive
- Oregano, dried
- Quinoa
- Rice, brown
- Sea salt
- Sunflower seeds
- Tomatoes, canned diced sodium-free
- Vinegar, apple cider
- Vinegar, balsamic

Essential Equipment

You won't need to purchase anything out of the ordinary to create the recipes in this book, but some dishes require certain tools to produce the best results or save time. You probably have some of the items listed, and the others can be purchased as you need them. Here are some tools and equipment to consider dusting off or adding to your kitchen arsenal:

Baking dishes: Baking dishes are used for roasting proteins, baking casseroles and desserts, and many other applications. Get an assortment that includes dishes with lids, metal dishes, and small ramekins.

Baking sheets: Metal or silicone baking sheets with a minimum 1-inch rim can be used for recipes ranging from desserts to meats. If you have space in your kitchen, get a full sheet and a half-sheet pan.

Cutting boards: Safe food preparation requires clean cutting boards designated for meats, vegetables, and seafood. If you have space in your kitchen, get boards in several sizes so you have the best one for each specific culinary task.

Food processor: This appliance is required for making nut butters, puréeing large batches, and preparing heaps of chopped vegetables. Look for a processor with a 10- to 12-cup capacity.

Good-quality blender: This tool is crucial for smoothies, soups, and grinding nuts. You don't need to spend a great deal of money on a blender, but find one that, at a minimum, can crush ice cubes easily.

High-quality kitchen knives: If you haven't already, using a perfectly balanced, finely honed, professional knife is a revelation. You cannot imagine the time and energy saved when you use a high-quality knife to chop, slice, and mince. Compare and hold several knives in the store to determine the most comfortable length, weight, and shape for your hand. You should also keep the knives sharpened for the best results.

Measuring cups and spoons: A recipe's result often depends on accurate measurements, so invest in a complete set of wet and dry measuring cups and measuring spoons ranging from ⅛ teaspoon to 1 tablespoon.

Nonstick cookware: A selection of pots, pans, and skillets in different sizes and depths can make your life easier in the kitchen. If you have to make a choice, get one large skillet, a larger stockpot for soups, and three saucepans (large, medium, and small).

Peeler and zester: These tools are convenient for preparing root vegetables and zesting citrus fruits. You can also use a peeler to make vegetable noodles.

Stainless steel bowls: You can never have too many bowls for recipe preparation.

Stainless steel is a preferred material for kitchen bowls because it is easy to clean and does not stain or rust.

Week 1 Meal Plan

MONDAY

Breakfast: Basil–Cherry Tomato Baked Egg (page 64)
Lunch: Fish Tacos with Root Vegetable Slaw (page 101)
Dinner: Tarragon Turkey with Navy Beans (page 116; double)

TUESDAY

Breakfast: Pecan Coconut Granola (page 54)
Lunch: Tarragon Turkey with Navy Beans (leftovers)
Dinner: Lamb Souvlaki (page 124) Lemon-Thyme Quinoa (page 82)

WEDNESDAY

Breakfast: Summer Egg White Frittata (page 63)
Lunch: Raw Pecan–Romaine Lettuce Wraps (page 87)
Dinner: Roasted Chicken with Asian Glaze (page 119)

THURSDAY

Breakfast: Coconut-Blueberry Drop Scones (page 57)
Lunch: Carrot-Turmeric Soup (page 93)
Dinner: Chili-Lime Tilapia (page 100) Cannellini Bean Pilaf (page 83)

FRIDAY

Breakfast: Almond-Oatmeal Smoothie
(page 129)

Lunch: Quinoa-Vegetable Ribbon Salad
(page 91)

Dinner: Pork Chops with Mediterranean
Vegetables (page 121; double)

SATURDAY

Breakfast: Lemon-Almond Meal Pancakes
(page 59)

Lunch: Pork Chops with Mediterranean
Vegetables (leftovers)

Dinner: Sautéed Shrimp with Veggie
Noodles (page 108)

SUNDAY

Breakfast: Wild Mushroom Breakfast Bake
(page 65)

Lunch: Avocado Stuffed with Salmon Salad
(page 110)

Dinner: Easy Chicken Chili (page 114)

SUGGESTED SNACKS

Pecan Coconut Granola (page 54)
Baked Plantain Crisps (page 75)
Mushroom Squash Pâté (page 72)
Peaches
Almonds

Week 1 Shopping List

DAIRY AND DAIRY ALTERNATIVES

- Almond milk, unsweetened, 2¼ cups
- Coconut milk, 1 cup
- Yogurt, plain low-fat, 2 tablespoons

FISH AND SHELLFISH

- Haddock fillets, 4 (4-ounce)
- Salmon, cooked, 12 ounces
- Shrimp, 16 to 20 count, 1 pound
- Tilapia fillets, 4 (6-ounce)

FRUITS AND VEGETABLES

- Apple, 1
- Asparagus, 1 bunch
- Avocados, 2
- Bell pepper, yellow, 1
- Blueberries, 1 pint
- Cabbage, red, 1 head
- Carrots, 2 pounds plus 4 carrots
- Celery stalks, 7
- Garlic, minced, 5 tablespoons
- Ginger, fresh, 1 (4-inch) piece
- Kale, 1 bunch
- Lemons, 6
- Lettuce, Romaine, 1 head
- Lime, 1
- Mushrooms, wild, 4 ounces
- Onions, red, 2
- Onions, sweet, 6
- Pomegranate, 1 (¼ cup arils)
- Scallions, 3
- Spinach, 4 ounces
- Summer squash, yellow, 2
- Tomatoes, cherry, 5 pints
- Tomatoes, grape, 2 pints
- Zucchini, 1½ pounds plus 4 zucchini

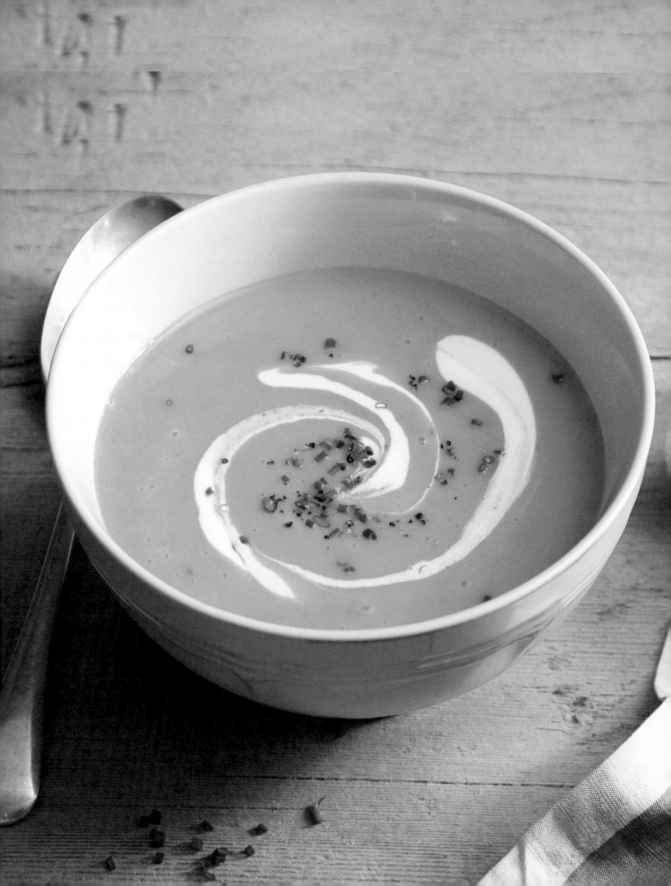

HERBS AND SPICES

- Basil, 1 small bunch
- Black pepper, freshly ground
- Cayenne pepper, pinch
- Chiles, dried, 3
- Chili paste, ½ teaspoon
- Chili powder, 2 tablespoons
- Cilantro, 1 small bunch
- Cinnamon, ground, 1⅛ teaspoons
- Coriander, ground, ½ teaspoon
- Cumin, ground, 4½ teaspoons
- Mint, 1 small bunch
- Oregano, 1 bunch
- Parsley, 1 bunch
- Sea salt
- Tarragon, 1 small bunch
- Thyme, 1 bunch
- Turmeric, ground, 2 teaspoons
- Vanilla extract, pure, ½ teaspoon

MEATS AND POULTRY

- Chicken breasts, boneless skinless, 2 (5-ounce)
- Chicken, drumsticks and thighs, 8 pieces
- Eggs, large, 19
- Lamb shoulder, 1 pound
- Pork chops, boneless, 32 ounces
- Turkey breast, boneless skinless, 32 ounces

OTHER

- Coconut, unsweetened shredded, 1¼ cups
- Edamame, frozen, ½ cup
- Olives, black, ½ cup sliced
- Sesame sauce, 2 tablespoons
- Tomatoes, sun-dried, ½ cup
- Tortillas, sprouted-grain, 4 (6-inch)

PANTRY ITEMS

- Almond flour, 2 cups
- Almonds, slivered, ¼ cup
- Arrowroot powder, ¼ cup
- Baking powder, 1 tablespoon
- Baking soda, ½ teaspoon
- Beans, cannellini, sodium-free, 1 (14.5-ounce) can
- Beans, navy, sodium-free, 3 (14-ounce) cans
- Broth, chicken, low-sodium, 1¼ cups
- Broth, vegetable, low-sodium, 8 cups
- Chia seeds, 1 tablespoon
- Chili paste, ½ teaspoon
- Coconut aminos, ¼ cup
- Coconut oil, ½ cup
- Hazelnuts, 1 cup
- Honey, raw, ½ cup
- Oats, rolled, ¼ cup
- Olive oil cooking spray
- Olive oil, extra-virgin, 1 tablespoon

- Pecans, ¼ cup
- Pistachios, ½ cup chopped
- Quinoa, dried, 4 cups
- Sunflower seeds, 1¼ cups
- Tomatoes, diced sodium-free, 1 (14.5-ounce) can
- Vinegar, apple cider, ¼ cup

Week 2 Meal Plan

MONDAY

Breakfast: Pecan Coconut Granola (page 54)
Lunch: Bean Caprese Salad (page 78)
Dinner: Lamb-Ginger Burgers (page 123; double)

TUESDAY

Breakfast: Wild Mushroom Breakfast Bake (page 65)
Lunch: Lamb-Ginger Burgers (leftovers)
Dinner: Millet-Stuffed Eggplant (page 94)

WEDNESDAY

Breakfast: Strawberry Peanut Butter Sprouted Wrap (page 56)
Lunch: White Bean–Cauliflower Soup (page 88)
Dinner: Haddock with Creamy Leeks (page 106)

THURSDAY

Breakfast: Basil–Cherry Tomato Baked Egg (page 64)
Lunch: Avocado Stuffed with Salmon Salad (page 110)
Dinner: Classic Nasi Goreng (page 95)

FRIDAY

Breakfast: Breakfast Nut and Seed Bars (page 55)
Lunch: Mediterranean Chickpea Toss (page 81)
Dinner: Roasted Chicken with Asian Glaze (page 119; double)

SATURDAY

Breakfast: Summer Egg White Frittata (page 63)
Lunch: Roasted Chicken with Asian Glaze (leftovers)
Dinner: Sautéed Shrimp with Veggie Noodles (page 108)

SUNDAY

Breakfast: Traditional French Toast with Peaches (page 62)
Lunch: Fish Tacos with Root Vegetable Slaw (page 101)
Dinner: Steak Diane Sauté (page 125)

SUGGESTED SNACKS

Breakfast Nut and Seed Bars (page 55)
Pear-Nutmeg Chips (page 79)
Oat Energy Balls (page 76)
Crudités with hummus
Grapes

Week 2 Shopping List

DAIRY AND DAIRY ALTERNATIVES

- Almond milk, unsweetened, ½ cup
- Coconut cream, ¼ cup
- Coconut milk, ¼ cup
- Mozzarella cheese, fresh, ½ cup shredded
- Yogurt, plain low-fat, 2 tablespoons

FISH AND SHELLFISH

- Haddock fillets, 4 (6-ounce) fillets plus 4 (4-ounce) fillets
- Salmon, cooked, 12 ounces
- Shrimp, 16 to 20 count, 1 pound

FRUITS AND VEGETABLES

- Asparagus, 1 bunch
- Avocados, 2
- Bell pepper, yellow, 1
- Cabbage, red, 1 head
- Carrots, 3
- Cauliflower, 2 heads
- Celery stalk, 1
- Cucumber, English, 1
- Eggplant, 2 small
- Garlic, minced, 5 tablespoons
- Ginger, fresh, 1 (6-inch piece)
- Kale, 1 bunch
- Leeks, 3
- Lemons, 4
- Mushrooms, button, 4 ounces
- Mushrooms, wild, 4 ounces
- Onion, red, 1
- Onions, sweet, 5
- Oranges, 2
- Peaches, 2
- Scallions, 5
- Spinach, 6 ounces
- Strawberries, ½ cup sliced
- Tomatoes, 4
- Tomatoes, cherry, 5 pints
- Zucchini, 1½ pounds plus 1 zucchini

HERBS AND SPICES

- Basil, 1 bunch
- Black pepper, freshly ground
- Chili paste, 1 teaspoon
- Cilantro, 1 small bunch
- Cinnamon, ground, 2½ teaspoons
- Cloves, ground, pinch
- Coriander, ground, ½ teaspoon
- Nutmeg, ground, ½ teaspoon
- Oregano, 1 small bunch
- Parsley, 1 small bunch
- Sea salt
- Thyme, 1 small bunch

MEATS AND POULTRY

- Bacon, uncured, 4 slices
- Beef rump steak, 1 pound
- Chicken, drumsticks and thighs, 16 pieces
- Eggs, large, 24
- Lamb, ground, 2 pounds

OTHER

- Almond extract, pure, ½ teaspoon
- Bread crumbs, panko, ¼ cup
- Bread, sprouted-grain, 8 slices
- Coconut, unsweetened shredded, 1 cup
- Millet, uncooked, 1 cup
- Mustard, Dijon, 1 tablespoon
- Olives, kalamata, ½ cup sliced
- Peanut butter, natural, ¼ cup
- Pumpkin seeds, ½ cup
- Sesame oil, ¼ cup
- Sesame sauce, 4 tablespoons
- Sesame seeds, ¼ cup
- Tortillas, sprouted-grain, 6 (6-inch)
- Vanilla extract, pure, 1 tablespoon

PANTRY ITEMS

- Almonds, chopped, 1 cup
- Beans, great northern or white, sodium-free, 1 (14.5-ounce) can
- Beans, white, sodium-free, 1 (7-ounce) can

- Broth, beef, low-sodium, ½ cup
- Broth, chicken, low-sodium, 8¾ cups
- Chia seeds, ¼ cup
- Chickpeas, sodium-free, 1 (14.5-ounce) can
- Coconut aminos, 5 tablespoons
- Coconut oil, 2 tablespoons
- Hazelnuts, 1¼ cups
- Honey, raw, 1 cup
- Oats, rolled, 2 tablespoons
- Olive oil cooking spray
- Olive oil, extra-virgin, 1 cup
- Pecans, chopped, 3 cups
- Peanut butter, natural, ¼ cup
- Rice, brown, 1½ cups
- Sunflower seeds, 1½ cups
- Vinegar, apple cider, ½ cup
- Vinegar, balsamic, 3 tablespoons

About the Recipes

The recipes in the following chapters use ingredients that are packed with nutrients and selected specifically to support a PCOS diet. Each recipe is clearly labeled with one or more of the following categories so you can choose foods based on factors important to your meal.

- **5-Ingredient:** These recipes use only 5 main ingredients or fewer. Pantry staples (page 42) are not counted among the ingredients.

- **30-Minute:** Recipes with this label need only 30 minutes (or less) to prepare—start to finish.
- **Dairy-Free:** These recipes do not contain any milk products.
- **Fertility Boost:** The ingredients in these recipes support and promote fertility and maintaining a healthy pregnancy.
- **Gluten-Free:** These recipes do not contain any gluten. This label flags dishes that are fine for people with celiac disease or those with gluten sensitivity.
- **Inflammation Fighter:** This label means the recipe's ingredients fight inflammation. These whole foods, usually, are high in antioxidants and phytonutrients.
- **Lower Calorie:** This label indicates that a dish is lower in calories and a good choice for those who have weight-loss or weight-maintenance goals.

3

Breakfast

Pecan Coconut Granola

30-Minute, Dairy-Free, Gluten-Free, Inflammation Fighter

Serves 12 Store-bought granola is usually packed with sugar and preservatives, so it is not a healthy way to start your day. Pecans are packed with antioxidants, including polyphenolic antioxidant ellagic acid, oleic acid, vitamin E, beta-carotene, and lutein—all of which help fight inflammation in the body. Pecans are also a fabulous source of folate, which is crucial for preventing birth defects. The other nuts and seeds included here are also rich in folate and healthy omega-3 fatty acids. Eat up and feel confident you're starting the day on a healthy note.

PREP: 5 minutes
COOK: 25 minutes

2 cups chopped pecans

1 cup unsweetened shredded coconut

1 cup sunflower seeds

1 cup hazelnuts

2 tablespoons melted coconut oil

2 tablespoons raw honey

½ teaspoon ground cinnamon

¼ teaspoon sea salt

1. Preheat the oven to 300°F.

2. Line a baking sheet with parchment paper and set aside.

3. In a large bowl, toss together the pecans, coconut, sunflower seeds, and hazelnuts.

4. In a small bowl, stir together the coconut oil, honey, cinnamon, and salt.

5. Add the coconut oil mixture to the nuts and stir until all ingredients are well coated.

6. Spread the mixture on the prepared sheet and bake for 20 to 25 minutes, stirring several times, until the granola is lightly browned.

7. Cool the granola completely and store in an airtight container for up to 1 week.

LOWER CALORIE TIP The coconut oil creates a slight crispness and golden color but it is not necessary if you want to cut calories and fat—about 20 calories and 3 grams of fat per serving. Just omit the oil and make the recipe as otherwise directed.

PER SERVING (¾ cup) Calories: 316; Carbohydrates: 10g; Glycemic Load: 2; Fiber: 5g; Protein: 5g; Sodium: 51mg; Fat: 31g

Breakfast Nut and Seed Bars

30-Minute, Dairy-Free, Fertility Boost, Gluten-Free, Inflammation Fighter, Lower Calorie

Makes 16 bars Almonds positively affect cholesterol levels and can improve insulin resistance because they are high in magnesium. Cinnamon has insulin-sensitizing properties so it is also an effective nutritional tool to improve insulin resistance. The seeds in these energy-packed bars provide folate, calcium, iron, and omega-3 fatty acids, creating a fertility-supporting grab-and-go breakfast or snack. You can double this recipe because the bars freeze very well. Individually wrapped, they last for up to 2 months.

PREP: 5 minutes
COOK: 20 minutes

1 cup chopped almonds

1 cup chopped pecans

½ cup sunflower seeds

¼ cup chia seeds

¼ cup sesame seeds

1 teaspoon ground cinnamon

Pinch ground cloves

½ cup raw honey

2 tablespoons coconut oil

1 teaspoon pure
vanilla extract

½ teaspoon pure
almond extract

1. Preheat the oven to 300°F.

2. Line a 9-by-13-inch baking dish with parchment paper and set aside.

3. In a large bowl, mix together the almonds, pecans, sunflower seeds, chia seeds, sesame seeds, cinnamon, and cloves.

4. Stir in the honey, coconut oil, vanilla, and almond extract until the mixture holds together. Firmly press the mixture into the prepared dish and bake for about 20 minutes, until golden brown.

5. Cool the squares and cut into 16 bars.

6. Refrigerate the squares in a sealed container for up to 2 weeks.

INFLAMMATION FIGHTER TIP Plant-based omega-3 fatty acids, known as alpha-linolenic acids (ALAs), are powerful anti-inflammatories. Nuts and seeds are great sources of omega-3s, but if you want to boost the amount in the bars, substitute flaxseed for the chia seeds because flaxseed has the highest quantity.

PER SERVING (1 bar) Calories: 191; Carbohydrates: 14g;
Glycemic Load: 5; Fiber: 3g; Protein: 4g; Sodium: 4mg; Fat: 15g

Strawberry Peanut Butter Sprouted Wrap

5-Ingredient, 30-Minute, Dairy-Free

Serves 2 Traditional peanut butter and jelly sandwiches are a staple in many households, so this healthier version should be a popular alternative. Natural peanut butter has absolutely no added sugar or preservatives and is high in fiber, protein, magnesium, vitamin E, and immune system–boosting vitamin B_6. This combination of nutrients ensures you stay full longer, especially when combined with sprouted-grain tortillas. Strawberries are one of the best fruit sources of antioxidants, and eating this sweet berry can reduce blood sugar elevations.

PREP: 10 minutes
COOK: none

2 (6-inch) sprouted-grain tortillas

¼ cup natural peanut butter

½ cup sliced strawberries

2 tablespoons rolled oats

2 tablespoons chopped hazelnuts

1. Place both tortillas on a clean work surface and spread 2 tablespoons peanut butter onto each, leaving about ½ inch at the edges.

2. Arrange the strawberry slices on the peanut butter and sprinkle each with oats and hazelnuts.

3. Fold the left and right edges of the tortillas into the center, laying the edges over the fruit. Starting at the edge closest to you, roll the tortilla away from you, creating a snug wrap.

4. Repeat with the second tortilla.

LOWER CALORIE TIP Omit the chopped hazelnuts to reduce calories by 45 and fat grams by 4. The oats add texture to this pretty grab-and-go breakfast option.

PER SERVING Calories: 299; Carbohydrates: 33g; Glycemic Load: 4; Fiber: 7g; Protein: 12g; Sodium: 143mg; Fat: 15g

Coconut-Blueberry Drop Scones

30-Minute, Dairy-Free, Fertility Boost, Gluten-Free, Inflammation Fighter, Lower Calorie

Serves 6 These tender berry-studded scones are rich in inflammation-fighting antioxidants, omega-3 fatty acids, and fiber from multiple ingredients, such as the almond flour, coconut, coconut oil, and blueberries. Honey contributes proteolytic enzymes and antioxidants that break down proteins and cellular waste and remove them from the body. The base recipe for these scones can be used to create other variations, such as lemon, dark chocolate chip, or cranberry.

PREP: 10 minutes
COOK: 20 minutes

1 cup almond flour

¼ cup unsweetened shredded coconut

½ teaspoon baking soda

Pinch sea salt

½ cup unsweetened almond milk

1 large egg

1 tablespoon raw honey

1 tablespoon melted coconut oil

¾ cup fresh blueberries

Olive oil cooking spray, for coating the skillet

1. In a large bowl, stir together the almond flour, coconut, baking soda, and sea salt until well mixed.

2. In a small bowl, whisk the almond milk, egg, honey, and coconut oil until blended.

3. Add the wet ingredients to the dry ingredients and whisk until the batter is smooth.

4. Stir in the blueberries.

5. Place a large skillet over medium-high heat and spray it lightly with cooking spray.

6. Drop the batter by tablespoons into the skillet. Cook the scones for about 4 minutes, until the bottoms are golden and bubbles form on the surface. Flip the scones and cook for about 2 minutes more, or until the other side is golden brown.

7. Repeat with the remaining batter.

COOKING TIP If you want a more uniform-looking scone, use a muffin pan instead of a skillet. Lightly grease the cups with cooking spray and bake the scones at 400°F for 15 minutes.

PER SERVING (4 scones) Calories: 111; Carbohydrates: 8g; Glycemic Load: 3; Fiber: 2g; Protein: 2g; Sodium: 42mg; Fat: 8g

Fresh Ginger Pear Muffins

30-Minute, Dairy-Free, Gluten-Free, Inflammation Fighter, Lower Calorie

---

Makes 12 muffins Muffins are a charming way to start your day especially when they are low in calories and saturated fat as well as packed with anti-inflammatory goodness. Ginger, almond flour, coconut oil, and honey are high in antioxidants, fiber, and nutrients that fight inflammation and support the digestive system. Make sure to source out oats produced in a gluten-free environment to avoid any issues with allergens.

PREP: 10 minutes
COOK: 20 minutes

1 cup almond flour

1 cup rolled oats

1½ teaspoons baking powder

¼ teaspoon salt

½ cup almond milk

⅓ cup melted coconut oil

2 eggs

2 tablespoons raw honey

1 tablespoon grated fresh ginger

1 teaspoon pure vanilla extract

1 pear, peeled, cored, and chopped

1. Preheat the oven to 400°F.

2. Line 12 muffin cups with paper wrappers and set the tray aside.

3. In a large bowl, stir together the almond flour, oats, baking powder, and salt until well combined.

4. In a medium bowl, whisk together the almond milk, coconut oil, eggs, honey, ginger, and vanilla until blended.

5. Add the wet ingredients to the dry ingredients and stir until just combined.

6. Fold in the pear and spoon the muffin batter into the prepared tray.

7. Bake until a toothpick inserted into one of the muffins comes out clean, about 18 to 20 minutes.

8. Cool on a wire rack and store extras in the refrigerator for up to 3 days.

> **INFLAMMATION FIGHTER TIP** Leave the skin on the pear for a considerable amount of soluble fiber. Fiber can support a healthy gut, which is crucial for fighting inflammation in the body.

PER SERVING (1 muffin) Calories: 147; Carbohydrates: 12g; Glycemic Load: 5; Fiber: 2g; Protein: 4g; Sodium: 73mg; Fat: 10g

Lemon–Almond Meal Pancakes

30-Minute, Dairy-Free, Fertility Boost, Gluten-Free, Inflammation Fighter, Lower Calorie

Serves 4 Pancakes are often placed on the "do not eat" list because, traditionally, they are made with white processed flour and served with buckets of butter and syrup. This version is made with almond flour, coconut oil, and nutrition-packed honey, and served with fresh fruit. Lemon juice and zest are packed with hormone-balancing vitamin C, so enjoying fluffy pancakes can support fertility.

PREP: 5 minutes
COOK: 15 minutes

1 cup almond flour

¼ cup fine arrowroot powder

1 tablespoon baking powder

Zest and juice of 1 lemon

¾ cup unsweetened almond milk

¼ cup coconut oil

2 tablespoons raw honey

Olive oil cooking spray, for coating the skillet

Fresh fruit, for serving

1. In a large bowl, stir together the flour, arrowroot powder, baking powder, and lemon zest until well mixed.

2. Whisk in the lemon juice, almond milk, coconut oil, and honey.

3. Place a large nonstick skillet over medium heat and coat it lightly with cooking spray.

4. With a ¼-cup measure, spoon pancakes into the skillet, about 4 per batch. Cook for about 3 minutes until bubbles start to break on the surface of the pancakes and flip. Cook the other side for about 1 minute. Transfer the pancakes to a plate and cover with a clean kitchen towel to keep warm. Repeat with the remaining batter.

5. Serve with your favorite fresh fruit.

INFLAMMATION FIGHTER TIP Make your own almond flour with a food processor rather than purchasing it. Use blanched almonds because the bran or hull of this nut contains enzyme inhibitors, which might cause inflammation in the body.

PER SERVING (2 pancakes) Calories: 227; Carbohydrates: 19g; Glycemic Load: 9; Fiber: 1g; Protein: 2g; Sodium: 302mg; Fat: 17g

Pepper and Egg Skillet

Dairy-Free, Fertility Boost, Gluten-Free, Inflammation Fighter, Lower Calorie

Serves 4 Jalapeño peppers are very low in calories and high in vitamins A and C, which help protect the body from free radicals and fight inflammation. Jalapeños also contain a phytochemical called capsaicin that inhibits substance P, which is associated with inflammatory processes. The more capsaicin in a pepper, the better it is for fighting inflammation. Jalapeños are considered a milder pepper, so if you want more capsaicin and like your food fiery hot, try habanero or serrano peppers.

PREP: 15 minutes
COOK: 25 minutes

2 tablespoons extra-virgin olive oil

1 sweet onion, thinly sliced

1 teaspoon minced garlic

1 red bell pepper, thinly sliced

1 green bell pepper, thinly sliced

1 jalapeño pepper, chopped

8 large eggs, beaten

Sea salt, for seasoning

Freshly ground black pepper, for seasoning

1. Preheat the oven to 375°F.

2. In a large ovenproof skillet over medium-high heat, heat the olive oil.

3. Add the onion and garlic and sauté for about 3 minutes, until softened.

4. Stir in the bell peppers and the jalapeño. Sauté for 5 minutes.

5. Pour in the eggs and cook for about 4 minutes, until the bottom is set, lifting the cooked eggs to let the uncooked eggs flow underneath.

6. Place the skillet in the oven and bake for about 10 minutes until the eggs are cooked through, puffy, and golden.

7. Season with salt and pepper and serve.

FERTILITY BOOST TIP Eggs are packed with a multitude of fertility-supporting nutrients, including choline, an important mineral for fetal development. The positive effects of adequate choline during pregnancy reach into adulthood. Add 1 cup blanched cauliflower florets to increase the choline in this hearty dish.

PER SERVING Calories: 234; Carbohydrates: 8g; Glycemic Load: 3; Fiber: 2g; Protein: 14g; Sodium: 168mg; Fat: 17g

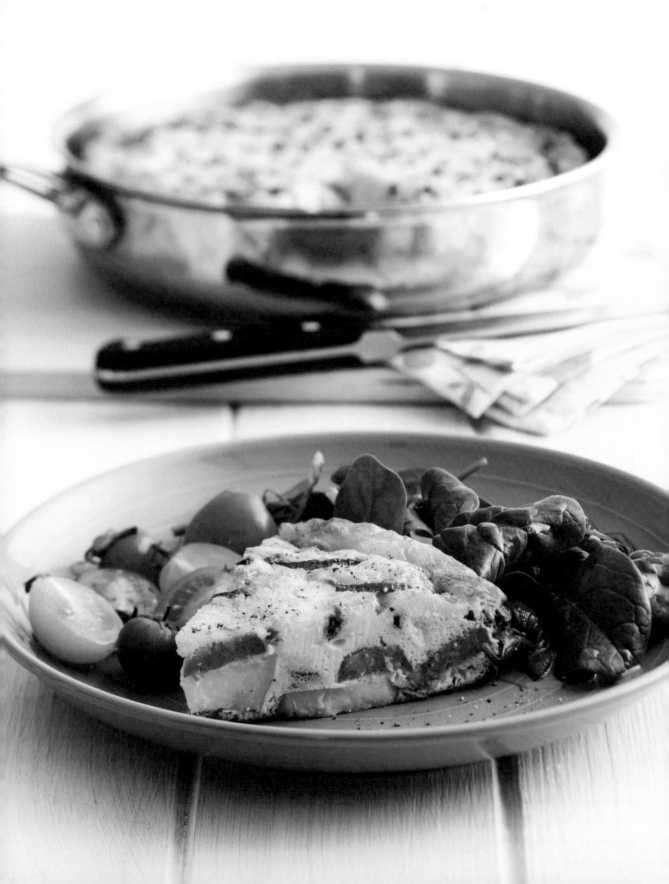

Traditional French Toast with Peaches

30-Minute, Dairy-Free, Fertility Boost, Gluten-Free, Inflammation Fighter, Lower Calorie

Serves 4 Peaches are low in calories and an excellent source of vitamins A and C and beta-carotene—all powerful antioxidants. Vitamin C plays an important role in hormonal health, regulation of the menstrual cycle, and ovarian function. Vitamin A helps follicles mature and supports better cervical fluid so conception is more likely. Beta-carotene supports regular ovulation and is a powerful inflammation fighter. If peaches are not in season, sweet and ripe, a couple of cups of fresh raspberries are also delicious.

PREP: 5 minutes
COOK: 12 minutes

4 large eggs

½ cup unsweetened almond milk

¼ cup freshly squeezed orange juice

2 teaspoons pure vanilla extract

1 teaspoon ground cinnamon

Olive oil cooking spray, for coating the skillet

8 slices sprouted bread

1 cup diced fresh peaches

1. In a large bowl, whisk the eggs, almond milk, orange juice, vanilla, and cinnamon until well blended.

2. Place a large nonstick skillet over medium heat and spray it lightly with cooking spray.

3. Dredge 4 bread slices in the egg mixture and shake off any excess. Arrange the soaked bread in the skillet so it does not overlap.

4. Cook for about 3 minutes, until the bottoms are lightly browned. Flip the bread and cook for about 3 minutes more, until browned. Transfer the French toast to a plate and cover with a clean kitchen towel to keep warm.

5. Lightly spray the skillet again and repeat with the remaining egg mixture and bread.

6. Serve with fresh peaches.

INGREDIENT TIP Sprouted-grain bread is made from wheat grains that have been sprouted and ground into flour. This extra step creates a product that is higher in protein, has about 25 percent fewer carbs, and has much less fat than whole-wheat bread. Sprouted grains also contain considerably less gluten.

PER SERVING (2 pieces) Calories: 233; Carbohydrates: 32g; Glycemic Load: 11; Fiber: 6g; Protein: 13g; Sodium: 211mg; Fat: 6g

Summer Egg White Frittata

30-Minute, Dairy-Free, Fertility Boost, Gluten-Free, Inflammation Fighter, Lower Calorie

Serves 4 Onion flavors this frittata, along with freshly minced garlic and a generous amount of colorful vegetables. The colors in the vegetables ensure they cover a broad range of inflammation-fighting antioxidants, such as lycopene (red), chlorophyll (green), beta-carotene (orange), and lutein (yellow). Add the quercetin in the onions and allicin in the garlic and you have a frittata that is anti-inflammation.

PREP: 5 minutes
COOK: 25 minutes

10 large egg whites

¼ teaspoon sea salt

¼ teaspoon freshly ground black pepper

1 tablespoon extra-virgin olive oil

½ sweet onion, chopped

1 teaspoon minced garlic

2 cups chopped kale

1 yellow bell pepper, chopped

¼ cup shredded carrot

1 cup halved cherry tomatoes

1. Preheat the oven to 375°F.

2. In a medium bowl, whisk the egg whites, salt, and pepper and set aside.

3. In a heavy ovenproof skillet over medium heat, heat the olive oil.

4. Add the onion and garlic and sauté for about 3 minutes, until softened.

5. Stir in the kale, bell pepper, and carrot. Cook for about 5 minutes, until the vegetables are tender.

6. Pour the seasoned egg whites into the skillet. Cook for about 3 minutes, until slightly set on the bottom.

7. Scatter the cherry tomatoes on top and place the skillet in the oven. Bake for about 10 minutes, uncovered, until set.

FERTILITY BOOST TIP This frittata uses only egg whites to keep calories at a minimum, but replacing half the whites with 4 whole eggs can increase nutrients such as calcium, vitamins A and D, and folate for additional support of a healthy reproductive system.

PER SERVING Calories: 109; Carbohydrates: 9g; Glycemic Load: 4; Fiber: 2g; Protein: 11g; Sodium: 305mg; Fat: 4g

Basil–Cherry Tomato Baked Egg

30-Minute, Dairy-Free, Gluten-Free, Inflammation Fighter, Lower Calorie

Serves 4 Baked eggs make a simple dish to start your day with high-quality protein to fuel your activities. Eggs are filled with vitamins, minerals, and antioxidants, including vitamins A, D, and E, lutein, and iron. The American Heart Association recommends eating one egg per day to take advantage of the nutritional benefits of this food. Boost the lutein content of this dish by adding one cup chopped kale to the sautéed vegetables.

PREP: 5 minutes
COOK: 25 minutes

Olive oil cooking spray, for coating the ramekins

1 tablespoon extra-virgin olive oil

1 zucchini, finely chopped

1 scallion, white and green parts, chopped

1 teaspoon minced garlic

2 cups halved cherry tomatoes

2 tablespoons chopped fresh basil leaves

Sea salt, for seasoning

Freshly ground black pepper, for seasoning

4 large eggs

1. Preheat the oven to 400°F.

2. Lightly coat 4 (8-ounce) ramekins with cooking spray, place them in a baking dish, and set aside.

3. In a large skillet over medium-high heat, heat the olive oil.

4. Add the zucchini, scallion, and garlic and sauté for about 3 minutes until softened.

5. Stir in the cherry tomatoes and basil and season the mixture with salt and pepper. Divide the tomato mixture among the ramekins.

6. Crack 1 egg into each ramekin. Bake for about 20 minutes, until the eggs are just set.

INFLAMMATION FIGHTER TIP For centuries, herbs have been considered medicinal in nature, beyond their contribution to culinary applications. Basil has powerful anti-inflammatory and antibacterial properties. Sage and rosemary would also be lovely in this dish and offer the same potent effects.

PER SERVING Calories: 118; Carbohydrates: 4g; Glycemic Load: 2; Fiber: 1g; Protein: 7g; Sodium: 81mg; Fat: 9g

Wild Mushroom Breakfast Bake

30-Minute, Dairy-Free, Fertility Boost, Gluten-Free, Inflammation Fighter, Lower Calorie

Serves 4 Mushrooms, tender asparagus, and spinach form a tasty base for baking sunny-side up eggs. Plan to make this dish a maximum of 48 hours after you purchase the asparagus because this vegetable is extremely perishable. Asparagus is an excellent source of vitamins A, C, and K, folate, zinc, and copper. It is considered a powerful anti-inflammatory because of those nutrients but also because of its saponins and flavonoids such as quercetin.

PREP: 10 minutes
COOK: 20 minutes

1 tablespoon extra-virgin olive oil

2 cups sliced wild mushrooms

½ cup chopped sweet onion

1 teaspoon minced garlic

2 cups chopped fresh spinach

2 cups (2-inch) asparagus pieces

4 large eggs

Sea salt, for seasoning

Freshly ground black pepper, for seasoning

2 teaspoons chopped freshly parsley leaves

1. Preheat the oven to 400°F.

2. In a large ovenproof skillet over medium-high heat, heat the olive oil.

3. Add the mushrooms, onion, and garlic and sauté for about 5 minutes, until softened.

4. Stir in the spinach and asparagus and sauté for 2 minutes.

5. With the back of a spoon, make 4 wells in the mixture and crack 1 egg into each well. Season the eggs with salt and pepper. Bake for about 10 minutes, until the eggs are set.

6. Serve topped with parsley.

FERTILITY BOOST TIP Mushrooms are the only vegetable source of vitamin D, and increasing vitamin D consumption can help regulate menstrual cycles and increase the number of mature follicles. Increase the amount of mushrooms to 2½ cups to boost the vitamin D content of this tasty breakfast choice.

PER SERVING Calories: 135; Carbohydrates: 7g; Glycemic Load: 3; Fiber: 2g; Protein: 10g; Sodium: 211mg; Fat: 9g

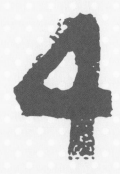

Snacks, Sides, and Appetizers

Spinach Tomato-Stuffed Mushrooms

5-Ingredient, 30-Minute, Dairy-Free, Gluten-Free, Inflammation Fighter, Lower Calorie

Serves 4 Mushrooms make the perfect container for fillings when you want to create attractive appetizers or snacks. Spinach, tomato, scallion, and garlic combine here to create a savory nutrient-rich blend that is beneficial for women with PCOS. To boost the health effects, add chopped nuts, such as almonds or pecans, and seeds like sunflower or pumpkin. These add omega-3 fatty acids and a satisfying crunch.

PREP: 10 minutes
COOK: 20 minutes

16 large white mushrooms, stemmed

2 teaspoons extra-virgin olive oil, divided

2 teaspoons minced garlic

1 cup chopped fresh spinach

½ cup chopped tomato

1 scallion, white and green parts, finely chopped

Sea salt, for seasoning

Freshly ground black pepper, for seasoning

1. Preheat the oven to 375°F.

2. Line a baking sheet with aluminum foil and place the mushrooms on the sheet, hollow-side up. Drizzle with 1 teaspoon olive oil and bake for 5 minutes to soften.

3. In a large skillet over medium-high heat, heat the remaining teaspoon olive oil.

4. Add the garlic and sauté for about 2 minutes until softened.

5. Add the spinach, tomato, and scallion to the skillet. Sauté for 4 minutes.

6. Season the filling with salt and pepper.

7. Spoon the filling into the mushroom caps and bake them for 5 minutes. Serve warm.

COOKING TIP If you want more filling in your mushrooms, use a spoon to scoop out some of the mushroom's flesh without breaking the cap. Chop the extra mushroom flesh and add it to the skillet with the garlic.

PER SERVING (4 stuffed caps) Calories: 50; Carbohydrates: 5g; Glycemic Load: 3; Fiber: 2g; Protein: 3g; Sodium: 45mg; Fat: 3g

Spice-Roasted Chickpeas

5-Ingredient, Dairy-Free, Gluten-Free, Inflammation Fighter, Lower Calorie

Serves 4 Roasted chickpeas are delightfully crisp and have a rich flavor that you might find slightly addictive. It is lucky that chickpeas are high in fiber, vitamins C and E, beta-carotene, manganese, folate, and copper. Chickpeas are highly effective for regulating blood sugar, as little as ½ cup per day for one week creates better blood sugar control. Try different types of seasoning on your chickpeas, such as dill, oregano, basil, coriander, or chili powder.

PREP: 10 minutes
COOK 45 minutes

2 cups canned sodium-free chickpeas, rinsed, drained, and patted dry with paper towels

2 teaspoons extra-virgin olive oil

½ teaspoon ground turmeric

¼ teaspoon ground cumin

Pinch sea salt

Pinch freshly ground black pepper

1. Preheat the oven to 375°F.

2. In a large bowl, toss together the chickpeas, olive oil, turmeric, cumin, salt, and pepper. Spread the chickpeas evenly on a baking sheet.

3. Bake for about 45 minutes until crisp and golden.

4. Cool the chickpeas completely and store them in a sealed container at room temperature for up to 5 days.

> **INFLAMMATION FIGHTER TIP** Turmeric is one of the best spices to fight inflammation in the body, but it can be an acquired taste. If you are not a fan of this spice, substitute cinnamon, ground ginger, or a pinch cayenne pepper because these spices are also anti-inflammatories.

PER SERVING Calories: 154; Carbohydrates: 22g; Glycemic Load: 8; Fiber: 6g; Protein: 7g; Sodium: 30mg; Fat: 4g

Mashed Cauliflower and Carrots

5-Ingredient, 30-Minute, Dairy-Free, Fertility Boost, Gluten-Free, Inflammation Fighter, Lower Calorie

Serves 4 Cauliflower is an exceptional fertility-boosting ingredient because it contains choline, a nutrient that can decrease the risk of birth defects, and DIM (diindolylmethane), a special phytonutrient that helps reduce estrogen dominance. Estrogen dominance can cause fertility issues in woman who have PCOS. Cauliflower is also rich in vitamins B_1, B_2, C, and K, as well as folate, fiber, omega-3 fatty acids, and manganese.

PREP: 10 minutes
COOK: 15 minutes

1 head cauliflower (about 3 pounds), cut into small florets

3 carrots, cut into 1-inch pieces

½ cup coconut milk

¼ teaspoon sea salt

¼ teaspoon ground nutmeg

Pinch freshly ground black pepper

1. Place a large pot of water over high heat and bring it to a boil.

2. Add the cauliflower and carrots. Blanch for about 10 minutes, until tender. Drain the vegetables and transfer to a food processor.

3. Add the coconut milk, salt, nutmeg, and pepper. Purée the vegetables until creamy and thick, about 2 minutes. Serve immediately.

FERTILITY BOOSTER TIP Carrots are very nutritious but swapping them for a couple of cups of cannellini beans ensures this side dish is very good for fertility. Cannellini beans are extremely high in folate, choline, and vitamin K. Note that adding the beans will add about 50 calories per serving.

PER SERVING Calories: 126; Carbohydrates: 15g; Glycemic Load: 7; Fiber: 7g; Protein: 6g; Sodium: 219mg; Fat: 6g

Carrot Ribbons with Dill

5-Ingredient, 30-Minute, Dairy-Free, Fertility Boost, Gluten-Free, Inflammation Fighter, Lower Calorie

Serves 4 For a spectacular-looking side dish, use different-colored carrots such as yellow, red, purple, and white. These different-hued varieties still have all the nutrients that make carrots a superfood. Lemon juice is rich in vitamin C and folate to support the reproductive system, and the fresh chopped dill is a great source of vitamin C and manganese. Compounds in dill can fight inflammation because they help oxidize molecules that would create damage in the body.

PREP: 15 minutes
COOK: 5 minutes

1 teaspoon extra-virgin olive oil

1½ pounds carrots, peeled and cut into long ribbons with a vegetable peeler

1 tablespoon freshly squeezed lemon juice

1 tablespoon chopped fresh dill

Sea salt, for seasoning

1. In a large skillet over medium heat, heat the olive oil.

2. Add the carrot ribbons and carefully sauté for about 5 minutes, until they are crisp-tender.

3. Toss the carrots with the lemon juice and dill and season with salt.

INFLAMMATION FIGHTER TIP Carrots contain a staggering amount of vitamin A—about 500 percent of the recommended daily amount is in one serving of this dish. The beta-carotene in carrots is converted into vitamin A in the liver. Beta-carotene and vitamin A are effective antioxidants and anti-inflammatories. Instead of dill, add 1 teaspoon ground turmeric to this pretty dish for an even more powerful inflammation-fighting combination.

PER SERVING Calories: 79; Carbohydrates: 16g; Glycemic Load: 4; Fiber: 5g; Protein: 2g; Sodium: 128mg; Fat: 2g

Mushroom Squash Pâté

Dairy-Free, Gluten-Free, Inflammation Fighter, Lower Calorie

Serves 8 Butternut squash has a velvety-smooth texture and rich golden color. The bright color of this vegetable comes from its high beta-carotene content, but butternut squash also has many other nutritional benefits. Butternut squash is high in vitamins A and C, folate, potassium, and omega-3 fatty acids, so including squash regularly fights inflammation and helps prevent birth defects. This recipe is just one tasty idea to help you do just that.

PREP: 10 minutes, plus 45 minutes cooling time
COOK: 12 minutes

2 tablespoons extra-virgin olive oil

2 cups shredded butternut squash

1 cup chopped button mushrooms

1 cup chopped shiitake mushrooms

½ sweet onion, finely chopped

1 teaspoon minced garlic

1 tablespoon chopped fresh thyme leaves

¼ teaspoon sea salt

Pinch freshly ground black pepper

1. In a large skillet over medium-high heat, heat the olive oil.

2. Add the squash, button and shiitake mushrooms, onion, and garlic. Sauté for about 10 minutes, until the vegetables are tender.

3. Add the thyme, salt, and pepper. Sauté for 2 minutes more. Transfer the mushroom mixture to a food processor and pulse for about 3 minutes until the mixture is smooth.

4. Transfer the mixture to a container and cool it to room temperature, about 45 minutes, before serving.

5. Cover and refrigerate the pâté for up to 1 week.

INFLAMMATION FIGHTER TIP Shiitake mushrooms contain a compound called ergothioneine that has the ability to inhibit oxidative stress. Use 2 cups shiitake mushrooms and omit the button mushrooms to increase the amount of this compound in each serving.

PER SERVING (½ cup) Calories: 63; Carbohydrates: 8g; Glycemic Load: 3; Fiber: 1g; Protein: 1g; Sodium: 76mg; Fat: 4g

Sweet Potato Hummus

30-Minute, Dairy-Free, Fertility Boost, Gluten-Free, Inflammation Fighter, Lower Calorie

Serves 4 Tahini—made from toasted, ground, hulled sesame seeds—is used in the cuisines of many countries, especially the Middle East. Sesame seeds are a stellar source of many important minerals such as copper, manganese, magnesium, calcium, and zinc. Copper is an often-overlooked mineral, but it is crucial for energy production in the body. An imbalance in copper and zinc can cause irregular ovulation. So, getting enough copper is very important. And this hummus is the way to do it!

PREP: 15 minutes
COOK: none

1½ cups mashed cooked sweet potato

½ cup canned chickpeas, drained and rinsed

¼ cup tahini

2 tablespoons extra-virgin olive oil

1 teaspoon minced garlic

¼ teaspoon ground cumin

¼ teaspoon ground coriander

Sea salt, for seasoning

Freshly ground black pepper

1. In a food processor, combine the sweet potato, chickpeas, tahini, olive oil, garlic, cumin, and coriander. Purée until smooth, scraping down the sides of the bowl as needed.

2. Season the hummus with salt and pepper. Keep covered and refrigerated for up to 1 week.

COOKING TIP Any type of cooked sweet potato works for this hummus, but baked sweet potatoes in their skins are the sweetest, fluffiest preparation. Bake the sweet potatoes at 400°F for 45 minutes and scoop the tender flesh from the crispy skin.

PER SERVING Calories: 251; Carbohydrates: 25g; Glycemic Load: 8; Fiber: 5g; Protein: 6g; Sodium: 52mg; Fat: 15g

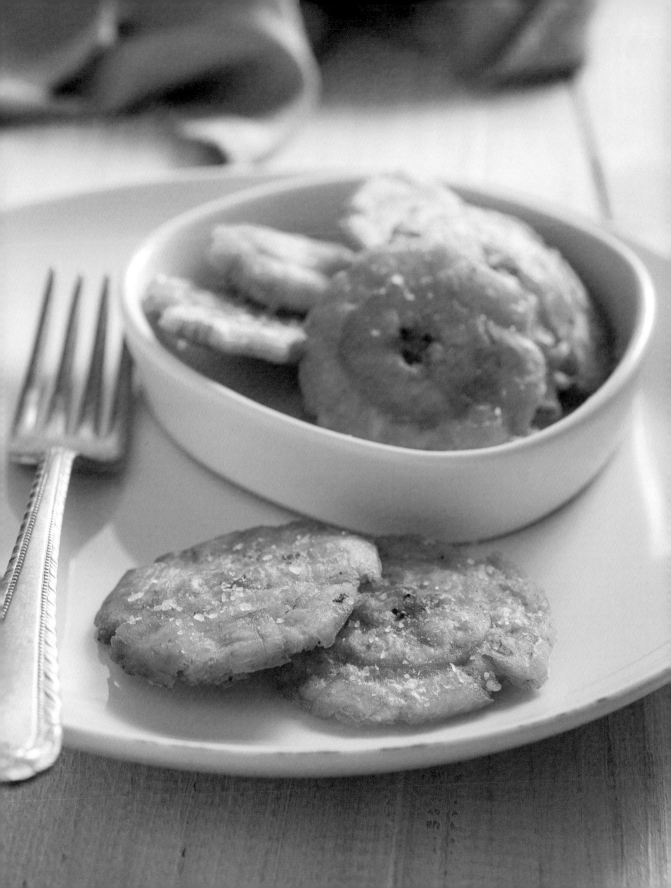

Baked Plantain Crisps

5-Ingredient, Dairy-Free, Gluten-Free, Inflammation Fighter, Lower Calorie

Serves 6 These crisps make a handy and healthy snack. Plantains are related to bananas but are usually treated like vegetables in culinary applications, and green plantains can only be eaten when cooked. Plantains are a good source of fiber, vitamins A, B complex, and C, potassium, iron, and magnesium. Cooking plantains actually improves their nutrition benefits, increasing vitamins A, B_6, and C as well as the potassium. Try savory spices such as cumin, coriander, and a pinch cayenne for a spicier snack.

PREP: 10 minutes
COOK: 30 minutes

1 pound green plantains, peeled and thinly sliced

2 tablespoons melted coconut oil

½ teaspoon ground cinnamon

¼ teaspoon ground nutmeg

Pinch cloves

Sea salt, for seasoning

1. Preheat the oven to 350°F.

2. Line a baking sheet with parchment paper and set aside.

3. In a large bowl, toss together the plantain slices, coconut oil, cinnamon, nutmeg, and cloves. Spread the plantain slices on the prepared sheet.

4. Bake the slices for about 30 minutes, until crisp, turning once halfway through.

5. Cool the slices completely and store them in a sealed container at room temperature for up to 3 days, or freeze for up to 1 month.

INGREDIENT TIP Plantains used to be a rare and exotic ingredient found only in specialty markets, but this fruit is now in almost every supermarket due to its popularity with foodies and those looking to eat a healthy diet. For these chips, look for plantains that are firm to the touch and slightly green so you can slice the fruit very thinly.

PER SERVING Calories: 130; Carbohydrates: 24g; Glycemic Load: 9; Fiber: 2g; Protein: 1g; Sodium: 19mg; Fat: 5g

Oat Energy Balls

Dairy-Free, Fertility Boost, Inflammation Fighter, Lower Calorie

Makes 12 balls Every ingredient in these incredible treats provides a big boost of energy, and they are perfect when you need an extra boost to get everything done. The best part of enjoying them is that you won't experience a blood sugar spike because the base is fiber-rich oats. Your blood sugar levels will stay stable all day, especially if you include high-fiber foods in your other meals. To make this dish gluten-free, you can use gluten-free rolled oats.

PREP: 10 minutes, plus 30 minutes chilling time
COOK: 0 minutes

2 cups rolled oats

½ cup sunflower seeds

¼ cup almond butter

¼ cup dried blueberries

2 tablespoons raw honey

½ teaspoon ground cinnamon

¼ teaspoon ground nutmeg

1. In a large bowl, stir together all the ingredients.

2. Roll the mixture into 1-inch balls and place them in a parchment paper-lined container.

3. Refrigerate the balls for about 30 minutes, until they become firm.

4. Keep covered and refrigerated for up to 1 week, or freeze for up to 1 month.

FERTILITY BOOST TIP Honey has been used as a treatment for infertility in Ayurvedic medicine for centuries and studies have shown that eating this sweet treat can stimulate the ovaries. Add 2 tablespoons wheat germ to add folate, which is crucial for healthy fetal development.

PER SERVING (1 ball) Calories: 181; Carbohydrates: 23g; Glycemic Load: 10; Fiber: 4g; Protein: 6g; Sodium: 1mg; Fat: 8g

Green Bean and Asparagus Pistachio Salad

30-Minute, Dairy-Free, Fertility Boost, Gluten-Free, Inflammation Fighter, Lower Calorie

Serves 4 Summer is the best time to get fresh green beans, but flash-frozen products also retain much of their nutritional value. Green beans are high in both fertility-boosting and anti-inflammatory nutrients, so they are an ideal choice for women with PCOS. They are also high in vitamins K and C, fiber, manganese, folate, and antioxidants such as chlorophyll, lutein, beta-carotene, violaxanthin, and neoxanthin.

PREP: 15 minutes
COOK: none

¼ cup extra-virgin olive oil

2 tablespoons apple cider vinegar

1 teaspoon chopped fresh thyme leaves

Sea salt, for seasoning

Freshly ground black pepper, for seasoning

1 pound green beans, blanched crisp-tender and cut into 2-inch pieces

1 pound asparagus, blanched crisp-tender and cut into 2-inch pieces

2 scallions, white and green parts, chopped

½ cup chopped pistachios

1. In a small bowl, whisk the olive oil, vinegar, and thyme. Season the dressing with salt and pepper.

2. In a large bowl, toss together the green beans, asparagus, scallions, and pistachios.

3. Add the dressing and toss to coat.

FERTILITY BOOST TIP Asparagus is a fabulous source of folate, and there are about 55 micrograms per serving in this salad. If you want to increase the folate content, use the asparagus raw because folate degrades when cooked.

PER SERVING Calories: 268; Carbohydrates: 17g; Glycemic Load: 6; Fiber: 8g; Protein: 8g; Sodium: 37mg; Fat: 21g

Bean Caprese Salad

5-Ingredient, 30-Minute, Gluten-Free, Inflammation Fighter, Lower Calorie

Serves 4 Women with PCOS should usually avoid most dairy products, so the fresh mozzarella in this Mediterranean-themed salad might be a surprise. Fresh mozzarella is low in calories, has 4 grams of fat per ounce, is high in vitamin A, calcium, and phosphorous, and is a good source of choline. If you use or make mozzarella with skim milk, you cut the fat in the cheese by 2 grams per ounce.

PREP: 15 minutes

COOK: none

2 cups canned Great Northern beans, drained and rinsed

2 cups halved cherry tomatoes

½ cup shredded fresh mozzarella cheese

½ cup fresh basil leaves

Sea salt, for seasoning

Freshly ground black pepper, for seasoning

2 teaspoons balsamic vinegar

1. In a large bowl, toss together the beans, tomatoes, mozzarella, and basil. Season the salad with salt and pepper.

2. Drizzle with the balsamic vinegar and serve.

> **INFLAMMATION FIGHTER TIP** Tomatoes are a stellar source of lycopene, an antioxidant that can combat inflammation in the brain. Adding 1 cup diced red bell peppers, also very high in lycopene, can increase the anti-inflammatory benefits of this salad.

PER SERVING Calories: 164; Carbohydrates: 27g; Glycemic Load: 8; Fiber: 11g; Protein: 13g; Sodium: 133mg; Fat: 1g

Pear-Nutmeg Chips

5-Ingredient, Dairy-Free, Gluten-Free, Inflammation Fighter, Lower Calorie

Serves 4 Pears are a splendid fruit often overlooked because apples are so popular. You might notice that this recipe uses unpeeled pears—the skin contains about four times the phytonutrients as the flesh. Flavonoids in pears (flavanols, flavan-3-ols, and anthocyanins) can improve insulin sensitivity. Pears are extremely high in fiber, vitamins C and K, and copper. Since this sweet fruit contains both soluble and insoluble fiber, it can help decrease the risk of type 2 diabetes and heart disease. Snack to your health.

PREP: 10 minutes

COOK: 45 minutes

4 pears, peel on, cored, and thinly sliced

1 teaspoon ground nutmeg

Sea salt, for seasoning

1. Preheat the oven to 300°F.

2. Line a baking sheet with parchment paper and arrange the pear slices with no overlap on the prepared sheet.

3. Sprinkle the slices with nutmeg and season very lightly with salt.

4. Bake the chips for about 45 minutes, turning once, until crisp and lightly golden brown.

5. Cool the chips and store them in a sealed container at room temperature for up to 5 days.

COOKING TIP Use pears that are just on the edge of being ripe so you can slice this fruit very thinly and create marvelously crisp chips. Ripe pears are too soft and roasting sweetens the unripe pears.

PER SERVING Calories: 86; Carbohydrates: 23g; Glycemic Load: 5; Fiber: 5g; Protein: 1g; Sodium: 26mg; Fat: 0g

Warm Sweet Potato Salad

5-Ingredient, Dairy-Free, Gluten-Free, Inflammation Fighter, Lower Calorie

Serves 4 Potato salad is often soaked in saturated fat, sodium, and high glycemic load carbs, but this dish is packed with healthy fiber-rich sweet potatoes and dressed in an anti-inflammatory apple cider vinegar and honey vinaigrette. The dressing is also flavored with fragrant thyme, which is high in vitamin C, iron, fiber, and manganese. Always use fresh thyme to boost nutrients in your meals because the volatile oils in herbs are sometimes depleted in the drying process.

PREP: 5 minutes, plus 10 minutes cooling time
COOK: 30 minutes

FOR THE DRESSING

2 tablespoons extra-virgin olive oil

¼ cup apple cider vinegar

1 tablespoon raw honey

1 teaspoon chopped fresh thyme leaves

FOR THE SALAD

1½ pounds sweet potatoes, peeled and cut into 1-inch chunks

1 tablespoon extra-virgin olive oil

1 scallion, white and green parts, chopped

Freshly ground black pepper, for seasoning

TO MAKE THE DRESSING

In a small bowl, whisk together all the ingredients. Set aside.

TO MAKE THE SALAD

1. Preheat the oven to 400°F.

2. Spread the sweet potato chunks on a baking sheet and drizzle with olive oil. Bake for about 30 minutes, until tender and lightly caramelized.

3. Cool for 10 minutes and transfer the sweet potatoes to a large bowl.

4. Add the dressing and the scallion to the potatoes and toss to combine.

5. Season with pepper and serve.

> **INGREDIENT TIP** Butternut squash, pumpkin, or yams could take the place of sweet potatoes if you want a slightly different taste, or combine all these wonderful choices for a spectacular salad.

PER SERVING Calories: 255; Carbohydrates: 35g; Glycemic Load: 15; Fiber: 5g; Protein: 3g; Sodium: 119mg; Fat: 10g

Mediterranean Chickpea Toss

30-Minute, Dairy-Free, Gluten-Free, Inflammation Fighter, Lower Calorie

Serves 4 This colorful salad might become a staple in your house because it is so delicious, nutritious, and energy packed and keeps you feeling full for hours. Cucumber might seem like a lightweight vegetable with respect to nutrition but it can hold its own among the other ingredients. Cucumbers are an excellent source of inflammation-busting phytonutrients, specifically cucurbitacin, lignans, and flavonoids. Cucumbers are also high in vitamin C, beta-carotene, and manganese—all powerful antioxidants.

PREP: 15 minutes
COOK: none

2 tablespoons balsamic vinegar

1 tablespoon extra-virgin olive oil

Sea salt, for seasoning

Freshly ground black pepper, for seasoning

2 cups canned chickpeas, drained and rinsed

2 tomatoes, chopped

1 English cucumber, chopped

½ red onion, chopped

½ cup sliced kalamata olives

2 tablespoons chopped fresh parsley leaves

1. In a small bowl, whisk the vinegar and olive oil. Season with salt and pepper and set aside.

2. In a large bowl, stir together the chickpeas, tomatoes, cucumber, onion, olives, and parsley.

3. Add the dressing and toss to coat.

INFLAMMATION FIGHTER TIP Many recipes can be enhanced with the addition of a cup or two of dark leafy greens, such as kale, spinach, or Swiss chard. These greens boost your intake of phytonutrients, antioxidants, and inflammation-fighting vitamins such as A and C.

PER SERVING Calories: 225; Carbohydrates: 29g; Glycemic Load: 10; Fiber: 8g; Protein: 9g; Sodium: 439mg; Fat: 9g

Lemon-Thyme Quinoa

5-Ingredient, 30-Minute, Dairy-Free, Gluten-Free, Inflammation Fighter, Lower Calorie

Serves 4 Quinoa is an incredibly versatile—and healing—ingredient. It is a seed from the same family as nutrition-packed spinach and Swiss chard. Quinoa is low on the glycemic index and a complete protein, which is unusual for a plant food. Quinoa is also incredibly rich in anti-inflammatory phytonutrients and nutrients such as quercetin, kaempferol, oleanic acid, omega-3 fatty acids, vitamin E, and saponins, and is high in fiber, so this dish can help regulate blood sugar.

PREP: 10 minutes
COOK: none

2 cups cooked quinoa

Zest and juice of 1 lemon

¼ cup chopped pistachios

2 teaspoons chopped fresh thyme leaves

Sea salt, for seasoning

Freshly ground black pepper, for seasoning

1. In a large bowl, stir together the quinoa, lemon zest and juice, pistachios, and thyme.

2. Season with salt and pepper.

INFLAMMATION FIGHTER TIP One of the best inflammation-busting nuts is walnuts, due, in part, to their high omega-3 fatty acid content. Use ¼ cup walnuts instead of pistachios here, or try almonds if you enjoy them best.

PER SERVING Calories: 199; Carbohydrates: 24g; Glycemic Load: 8; Fiber: 4g; Protein: 7g; Sodium: 32mg; Fat: 9g

Cannellini Bean Pilaf

30-Minute, Dairy-Free, Fertility Boost, Gluten-Free, Inflammation Fighter, Lower Calorie

Serves 4 There is only ½ cup edamame in this nutritious pilaf, but even that amount has as much fiber as four slices of whole-wheat bread and as much iron as one 4-ounce chicken breast. Edamame is also extremely high in plant protein, which promotes fertility. Add a couple of stalks of celery and you can boost the inflammation-fighting capacity of this dish. Celery can help decrease blood pressure and lower bad cholesterol.

PREP: 10 minutes
COOK: 15 minutes

1 tablespoon extra-virgin olive oil

2 celery stalks, chopped

1 sweet onion, chopped

1 carrot, finely chopped

1 teaspoon minced garlic

2 cups canned cannellini beans, drained and rinsed

½ cup edamame

1 teaspoon ground cumin

2 tablespoons chopped fresh parsley leaves

1 tablespoon chopped fresh oregano leaves

1. In a large skillet over medium-high heat, heat the olive oil.

2. Add the celery, onion, carrot, and garlic. Sauté for about 7 minutes, until tender.

3. Stir in the beans, edamame, and cumin. Sauté for about 5 minutes more, until warmed through.

4. Stir in the parsley and oregano and serve.

FERTILITY BOOST TIP Add 1 cup cauliflower florets or a small bunch of asparagus to the pilaf to add choline or folate to the dish. Sauté the vegetables along with the celery and carrots until tender.

PER SERVING Calories: 173; Carbohydrates: 25g; Glycemic Load: 7; Fiber: 10g; Protein: 10g; Sodium: 32mg; Fat: 4g

5

Vegetarian and Vegan Entrées

Sweet Potato–Cabbage Casserole

5-Ingredient, Dairy-Free, Fertility Boost, Gluten-Free, Inflammation Fighter, Lower Calorie

Serves 6 Cabbage is a good choice for a PCOS diet because it contains DIM (diindolylmethane), a phytonutrient that can help prevent fibroids and endometriosis (contributing factors of infertility) and assists estrogen metabolism. Cabbage is rich in vitamin C and an amino acid called glutamine, believed to strengthen the immune system and fight inflammation.

PREP: 10 minutes
COOK: 25 minutes

2 tablespoons extra-virgin olive oil

½ sweet onion, thinly sliced

6 cups finely shredded cabbage

2 cups mashed cooked sweet potato

½ cup unsweetened almond milk

¼ cup chopped fresh parsley leaves

Sea salt, for seasoning

Freshly ground black pepper, for seasoning

1. In a large skillet over medium-high heat, heat the olive oil.

2. Add the onion and sauté for about 3 minutes until softened.

3. Stir in the cabbage. Sauté for about 10 minutes, until tender.

4. Stir in the sweet potato, almond milk, and parsley until well combined. Season with salt and pepper. Cook for about 10 minutes, until the sweet potato mixture is piping hot. Serve immediately.

COOKING TIP This dish freezes well, so make a double batch to have on hand when you want a quick, immune-supporting meal on a busy evening. Thaw the casserole in the refrigerator during the day and pop it into a 375°F oven for about 45 minutes, or until heated through.

PER SERVING Calories: 129; Carbohydrates: 20g; Glycemic Load: 7; Fiber: 5g; Protein: 3g; Sodium: 52mg; Fat: 5g

Raw Pecan–Romaine Lettuce Wraps

30-Minute, Dairy-Free, Fertility Boost, Gluten-Free, Inflammation Fighter, Lower Calorie

Serves 4 Lettuce is often considered a throwaway ingredient, with no real nutritional contribution to a dish. However, romaine lettuce is extremely low in calories and packed with PCOS-fighting nutrients such as chromium. Chromium supports weight-loss goals because it helps control hunger and cravings. Chromium fights insulin resistance as an element of a glucose tolerance factor. This factor makes insulin more effective, which, in turn, maintains normal blood glucose levels. Nothing to throw away here!

PREP: 20 minutes
COOK: none

2 cups pecans

½ cup sun-dried tomatoes

1 teaspoon ground cumin

1 teaspoon chopped fresh cilantro leaves

8 large romaine lettuce leaves, stemmed

2 tablespoons Fresh Chile Pesto (page 143)

1. In a blender, combine the pecans, tomatoes, cumin, and cilantro. Pulse until blended and finely chopped.

2. Arrange the romaine lettuces leaves on a clean work surface and spread each leaf with the pesto.

3. Divide the pecan filling among the leaves and roll them up like burritos.

FERTILITY BOOST TIP Add ½ cup black beans to the pecan filling. This legume is rich in phytoestrogen to support the maturation of healthy eggs. Lentils are also a fabulous addition for increased amounts of folate.

PER SERVING (2 filled leaves) Calories: 241; Carbohydrates: 15g; Glycemic Load: 4; Fiber: 5g; Protein: 6g; Sodium: 172mg; Fat: 20g

White Bean–Cauliflower Soup

30-Minute, Dairy-Free, Fertility Boost, Gluten-Free, Inflammation Fighter, Lower Calorie

Serves 6 Cauliflower is an ideal vegetable to purée into a smooth silky soup, and the white beans enhance the comforting texture. If you want a more colorful soup, cauliflower comes in orange, green, and vibrant purple as well. The purple cauliflower is actually healthier than the white, with an abundance of the antioxidant anthocyanin, which is instrumental in reducing inflammation. If you decide to make a purple soup, you can still use all the other ingredients with no changes.

PREP: 10 minutes
COOK: 20 minutes

1 tablespoon extra-virgin olive oil

1 sweet onion, chopped

1 teaspoon minced garlic

8 cups low-sodium chicken broth

2 cauliflower heads, cut into florets

1 (7-ounce) can sodium-free white beans, drained and rinsed

½ teaspoon ground nutmeg

Sea salt, for seasoning

Freshly ground black pepper, for seasoning

1. In a large saucepan over medium-high heat, heat the olive oil.

2. Add the onion and garlic and sauté for about 3 minutes, until softened.

3. Stir in the broth, cauliflower, beans, and nutmeg. Bring the soup to a boil. Reduce the heat to low and simmer for about 15 minutes, until the cauliflower is tender.

4. Transfer the soup to a food processor and purée until velvety smooth.

5. Transfer the soup back to the saucepan to warm, and season with salt and pepper.

COOKING TIP Boiling your own beans is easy, and they keep for up to a week in the refrigerator for your various recipe needs. Pick through the dried beans for rocks and other imperfections, rinse, and simmer them in water for about 1 hour until tender.

PER SERVING Calories: 173; Carbohydrates: 23g; Glycemic Load: 11; Fiber: 9g; Protein: 13g; Sodium: 171mg; Fat: 5g

Squash-Lentil Bowl

30-Minute, Dairy-Free, Fertility Boost, Gluten-Free, Inflammation Fighter, Lower Calorie

Serves 4 Lentils are a simple ingredient that packs a significant nutritional punch. They contain molybdenum, folate, fiber, copper, protein, and iron. The soluble fiber in lentils can help stabilize blood sugar because it is a slow-burn energy source. The squash and green beans are also high in fiber, so enjoying this dish for lunch can help keep you going for the rest of the day with no need to snack.

PREP: 10 minutes
COOK: 20 minutes

1 teaspoon extra-virgin olive oil

1 sweet onion, chopped

2 teaspoon minced garlic

½ butternut squash, cut into 1-inch cubes, cooked

2 cups canned sodium-free lentils, drained and rinsed

2 tomatoes, diced

1 cup blanched (1-inch) green beans pieces

2 scallions, white and green parts, thinly sliced

1. In a large skillet over medium-high heat, heat the olive oil.

2. Add the onion and garlic and sauté for about 3 minutes, until softened.

3. Stir in the squash, lentils, tomatoes, and green beans. Cook for about 15 minutes until heated through.

4. Serve topped with scallions.

FERTILITY BOOST TIP Lentils are a wonderful choice for those seeking to boost fertility because they are very high in iron. Iron deficiencies can cause poor egg health as well as anovulation (lack of ovulation). This issue can decrease the chances of pregnancy by as much as 60 percent. Aim for about 27 milligrams of iron per day to maintain a healthy level.

PER SERVING Calories: 196; Carbohydrates: 35g; Glycemic Load: 12; Fiber: 10g; Protein: 11g; Sodium: 11mg; Fat: 2g

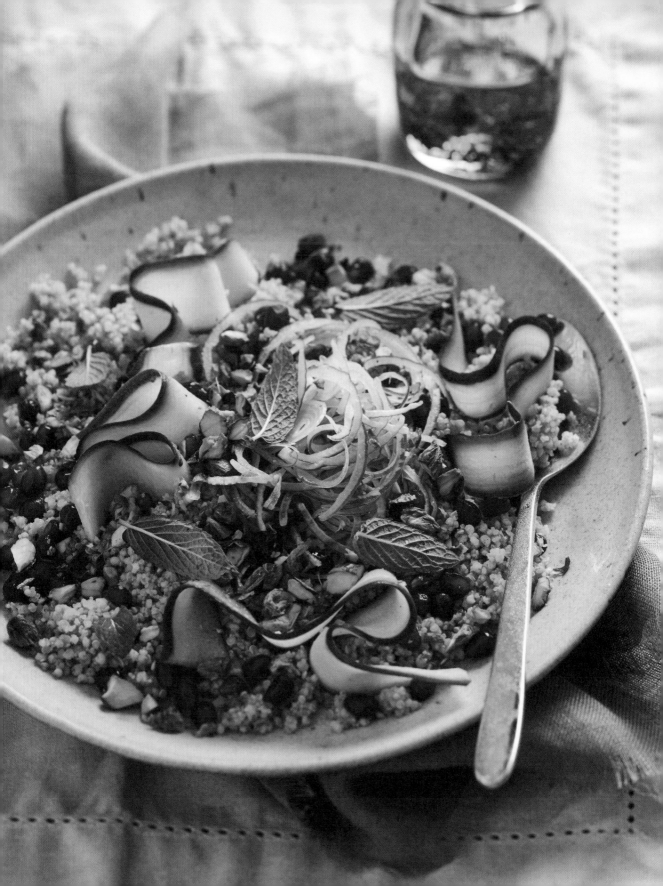

Quinoa-Vegetable Ribbon Salad

30-Minute, Dairy-Free, Fertility Boost, Gluten-Free, Inflammation Fighter

Serves 4 Sunflower seeds are sometimes avoided because they are high in calories, but this factor should not deter you from including these PCOS-fighting seeds in your meals. Sunflower seeds are a stellar source of vitamins B_2 and B_6, magnesium, and zinc. Vitamin B_2 is needed to reuse an important antioxidant in the body called glutathione. Vitamin B_6 deficiency can increase the effects of inflammation, so eat foods rich in this vitamin, like the sunflower seeds in this pretty and powerful presentation.

PREP: 25 minutes
COOK: none

FOR THE DRESSING

3 tablespoons extra-virgin olive oil

2 tablespoons freshly squeezed lemon juice

1 tablespoon raw honey

1 teaspoon minced garlic

1 teaspoon coconut aminos

FOR THE SALAD

2 cups cooked quinoa

1 zucchini, cut into ribbons with a vegetable peeler

½ red onion, thinly sliced

¼ cup pomegranate arils (seeds)

¼ cup chopped pistachios

2 tablespoons sunflower seeds

Fresh mint leaves, for garnish

TO MAKE THE DRESSING

In a small bowl, whisk together all the ingredients. Set aside.

TO MAKE THE SALAD

1. In a large bowl, toss the quinoa and half the dressing until well mixed.

2. Top the quinoa with the zucchini, onion, pomegranate arils, pistachios, and sunflower seeds.

3. Drizzle with the remaining dressing and garnish with mint.

FERTILITY BOOST TIP Pomegranate is a good source of vitamin C, which improves hormone levels and reduces the risk of chromosomal damage, and can reduce the risk of miscarriage. Eat pomegranate several times a week for good health and fertility.

PER SERVING Calories: 318; Carbohydrates: 29g; Glycemic Load: 11; Fiber: 5g; Protein: 8g; Sodium: 9mg; Fat: 20g

Southwestern Quinoa Skillet

30-Minute, Dairy-Free, Fertility Boost, Gluten-Free, Inflammation Fighter, Lower Calorie

Serves 4 Black beans don't seem to fall into that group of high-antioxidant colorful foods because they are not brightly hued. However, the beans' black color means they are rich in flavonoids such as delphinidin, petunidin, malvidin, kaempferol, and quercetin. Black beans are high in folate, copper, protein, and iron to support fertility. Eat three servings (about ½ cup) of legumes, such as black beans, at least three times per week.

PREP: 10 minutes
COOK: 20 minutes

2 teaspoons extra-virgin olive oil

½ jalapeño pepper, minced

2 teaspoons minced garlic

1 teaspoon ground cumin

½ teaspoon chili powder

2 cups cooked quinoa

1 cup canned sodium-free black beans, drained and rinsed

1 cup edamame

1 cup chopped tomato

Juice of 1 lime

1. In a large skillet over medium-high heat, heat the olive oil.

2. Add the jalapeño, garlic, cumin, and chili powder. Sauté for 3 minutes.

3. Stir in the quinoa, black beans, edamame, and tomato. Cook for about 15 minutes until heated through.

4. Stir in the lime juice and serve.

FERTILITY BOOST TIP Folic acid is one of the most important vitamins when considering fertility and pregnancy because a deficiency can increase the risk of neural tube defects, preterm labor, and pregnancy complications. Edamame is a stellar source of folic acid, with about 90 micrograms per ¼ cup. Add 1 cup shredded spinach to this dish to double your intake.

PER SERVING Calories: 231; Carbohydrates: 35g; Glycemic Load: 13; Fiber: 8g; Protein: 11g; Sodium: 11g; Fat: 6g

Carrot-Turmeric Soup

Dairy-Free, Gluten-Free, Inflammation Fighter, Lower Calorie

Serves 6 Carrots are best at summer's peak when they are sweet, bright, and, preferably, right out of the garden. Carrots are an incredible source of vitamins A, C, and K, fiber, potassium, and many inflammation-fighting phytonutrients, such as beta-carotene, polyacetylenes, and anthocyanins. Do not over-boil this soup; remove it from the heat as soon as the carrots are tender because prolonged boiling depletes their nutritional content.

PREP: 10 minutes
COOK: 25 minutes

1 tablespoon extra-virgin olive oil

1 sweet onion, chopped

1 teaspoon grated fresh ginger

1 teaspoon minced garlic

8 cups low-sodium vegetable broth

2 pounds carrots, chopped

2 teaspoons ground turmeric

Sea salt, for seasoning

1 cup coconut milk

2 teaspoons chopped fresh thyme leaves

1. In a large saucepan over medium-high heat, heat the olive oil.

2. Add the onion, ginger, and garlic and sauté for about 3 minutes, until softened.

3. Stir in the broth, carrots, and turmeric. Bring the soup to a boil. Reduce the heat to low and simmer for about 15 minutes, until the vegetables are tender.

4. Transfer the soup to a food processor and pulse until very smooth. Return the soup to the saucepan and season with salt.

5. Serve each bowl drizzled with a generous pour of coconut milk and top with the thyme.

INFLAMMATION FIGHTER TIP Turmeric contains an active compound called curcumin, which has anti-inflammatory and antioxidant properties. Curcumin shuts off the production of two inflammation-causing enzymes, COX-2 and 5-LOX, and shuts off inflammatory pathways. Increase the amount of turmeric in this recipe by 1 teaspoon to increase the effect even further.

PER SERVING Calories: 173; Carbohydrates: 21g; Glycemic Load: 5; Fiber: 5g; Protein: 2g; Sodium: 432mg; Fat: 10g

Millet-Stuffed Eggplant

Dairy-Free, Fertility Boost, Gluten-Free, Inflammation Fighter, Lower Calorie

Serves 4 Stuffed vegetables make a satisfying meal and eggplant is perfect for filling with toasty millet, sweet tomatoes, and crunchy pumpkin seeds. Eggplant contains phenolic compounds, specifically chlorogenic acid, and an antioxidant that is one of the strongest free-radical fighters. Pumpkin seeds are extremely high in zinc, an essential mineral for cell division in the embryonic stage of pregnancy. Zinc also helps ensure healthy egg development.

PREP: 10 minutes
COOK: 23 minutes

1 tablespoon extra-virgin olive oil

½ sweet onion, chopped

2 teaspoons minced garlic

2 cups cooked millet

2 tomatoes, diced

1 cup shredded fresh spinach

½ cup pumpkin seeds

1 tablespoon chopped fresh basil leaves

1 tablespoon freshly squeezed lemon juice

½ teaspoon ground coriander

Sea salt, for seasoning

Freshly ground black pepper, for seasoning

2 small eggplants, halved, flesh scooped out to within ½ inch of the skin, flesh reserved for another use, such as a pasta sauce or dip

1. Preheat the oven to 400°F.

2. In a large skillet over medium-high heat, heat the olive oil.

3. Add the onion and garlic and sauté for about 3 minutes, until softened.

4. Stir in the millet, tomatoes, spinach, pumpkin seeds, basil, lemon juice, and coriander. Season with salt and pepper. Spoon the filling into the eggplant halves and place them on a baking sheet.

5. Bake for about 20 minutes until the eggplant is tender and the filling is heated through.

> **FERTILITY BOOST TIP** Millet is an underused grain that helps balance insulin levels, which keeps hormones in balance. Millet is extremely rich in fiber, vitamins E and B complex, and iron. Mix millet with quinoa or oats to create a nutritional powerhouse.

PER SERVING Calories: 194; Carbohydrates: 29g; Glycemic Load: 13; Fiber: 3g; Protein: 6g; Sodium: 25mg; Fat: 6g

Classic Nasi Goreng

Dairy-Free, Fertility Boost, Gluten-Free, Inflammation Fighter, Lower Calorie

Serves 4 Nasi goreng is Indonesian fried rice, a dish created to use up leftover rice rather than throw it away. Brown rice is a complex carbohydrate that is extremely high in fiber, vitamins B and E, manganese, selenium, phosphorous, and magnesium. Brown rice helps stabilize insulin and blood sugar levels, balances hormones, and is crucial for cellular reproduction. The carrot and onion increase the fiber content and effects of this nutrient.

PREP: 15 minutes
COOK: 18 minutes

1 tablespoon extra-virgin olive oil

1 carrot, finely chopped

½ cup chopped onion

2 teaspoons grated fresh ginger

2 teaspoons minced garlic

3 cups cooked brown rice

1 tablespoon coconut aminos

2 large eggs, beaten

1 scallion, white and green parts, thinly sliced on a bias

1. In a large skillet over medium-high heat, heat the olive oil.

2. Add the carrot, onion, ginger, and garlic and sauté for about 5 minutes, until softened.

3. Stir in the brown rice and coconut aminos. Sauté for about 10 minutes more until the rice is heated through.

4. Move the rice to the side of the skillet and pour the eggs into the skillet. Scramble the eggs until your desired doneness and mix them into the rice.

5. Serve topped with scallions.

INGREDIENT TIP Coconut aminos is a great choice for anyone trying to avoid soy products or those wanting to limit sodium intake. This tasty condiment can be found in most grocery stores in the organic section or Asian foods section.

PER SERVING Calories: 245; Carbohydrates: 36g; Glycemic Load: 16; Fiber: 3g; Protein: 8g; Sodium: 138mg; Fat: 7g

Broccolini–Swiss Chard Sauté

5-Ingredient, 30-Minute, Dairy-Free, Fertility Boost, Gluten-Free, Inflammation Fighter, Lower Calorie

Serves 4 Eating your greens has never been so good for you. Broccolini is a wonderful source of folic acid, vitamin C, and iron. Folic acid, a nutrient that has been proven essential to a successful, healthy pregnancy, helps prevent disorders such as spina bifida. Folic acid also supports egg development. Vitamin C is critical for ovulation because the ovaries need this vitamin to mature the eggs. Iron builds a healthy endometrial lining, which ensures that the zygote can attach effectively to the uterus and stays attached.

PREP: 10 minutes
COOK: 7 minutes

1 tablespoon extra-virgin olive oil

¼ onion, chopped

2 teaspoons minced garlic

4 cups chopped broccolini, about 3 bunches

2 cups chopped Swiss chard

Zest and juice of 1 lemon

Sea salt, for seasoning

Freshly ground black pepper, for seasoning

1. In a large skillet over medium-high heat, heat the olive oil.

2. Add the onion and garlic and sauté for about 2 minutes, until tender.

3. Add the broccolini and Swiss chard. Sauté for about 5 minutes, until the broccolini is bright green and crisp-tender.

4. Remove the skillet from the heat and stir in the lemon zest and juice.

5. Season with salt and pepper and serve immediately.

INFLAMMATION FIGHTER TIP Instead of onion, substitute ¼ cup thinly sliced shallots, which are packed with vitamins, minerals, and antioxidants in higher quantities than the same quantity of onion.

PER SERVING Calories: 69; Carbohydrates: 8g; Glycemic Load: 4; Fiber: 3g; Protein: 3g; Sodium: 82mg; Fat: 4g

Cauliflower Fritters

30-Minute, Dairy-Free, Fertility Boost, Gluten-Free, Inflammation Fighter, Lower Calorie

Makes 8 fritters Fritters are really just vegetable burgers in a slightly smaller patty or shaped into ovals for a different presentation. This recipe contains two types of seeds that are perfect for both fertility boosting and fighting damaging inflammation. It is important to use raw seeds because they retain their nutrients and provide essential fatty acids and zinc, which can deteriorate when the seeds are heated.

PREP: 15 minutes
COOK: 15 minutes

4 cups finely chopped cauliflower, in a food processor if possible

1 carrot, grated

2 eggs

½ cup almond flour

¼ cup raw unsalted sunflower seeds

1 tablespoon sesame seeds

1 tablespoon chopped fresh parsley

2 teaspoons freshly squeezed lemon juice

1 teaspoon chopped fresh thyme

¼ teaspoon sea salt

¼ teaspoon freshly ground black pepper

Pinch cayenne pepper

2 tablespoons extra-virgin olive oil

1. In a large bowl, combine the cauliflower, carrot, eggs, almond flour, sunflower seeds, sesame seeds, parsley, lemon juice, thyme, sea salt, black pepper, and cayenne until the mixture is well mixed and holds together when pressed.

2. Roll the mixture into eight equal pieces, pressing them into patties about ½ inch thick.

3. Place a large skillet over medium-high heat and add the olive oil.

4. Panfry four fritters, until golden on both sides turning once, about 3 minutes per side.

5. Repeat with the remaining fritters.

6. Serve warm.

FERTILITY BOOST TIP Flaxseed can take the place of the sesame seed in this recipe in the same amount. Flaxseeds are very high in protein and omega-3 fatty acids, which are important nutrients for fertility.

PER SERVING (2 fritters) Calories: 254; Carbohydrates: 12g; Glycemic Load: 3; Fiber: 6g; Protein: 7g; Sodium: 186mg; Fat: 21g

6

Fish and Seafood Entrées

Chili-Lime Tilapia

5-Ingredient, 30-Minute, Dairy-Free, Fertility Boost, Gluten-Free, Inflammation Fighter, Lower Calorie

Serves 4 You won't find a great deal of cinnamon in this rub, but even a small amount mellows the chili powder and adds a lovely complexity to the flavor. Cinnamon has a positive impact for women with PCOS in several ways. An active ingredient in cinnamon called hydroxychalcone increases insulin sensitivity. Cinnamon can also affect the speed at which food leaves the stomach, so post-meal blood sugar spikes are unlikely.

PREP: 10 minutes
COOK: 10 minutes

1 teaspoon chili powder

½ teaspoon ground cinnamon

¼ teaspoon ground coriander

4 (6-ounce) tilapia fillets, patted dry

1 teaspoon extra-virgin olive oil

Juice of 1 lime

1. Preheat the oven to 400°F.

2. Line a small baking sheet with aluminum foil and set aside.

3. In a small bowl, stir together the chili powder, cinnamon, and coriander until well mixed.

4. Rub the spice mixture onto both sides of the fish and place them on the prepared sheet.

5. Drizzle the fish with olive oil and lime juice.

6. Bake for about 10 minutes, until the tilapia flakes easily with a fork.

> **FERTILITY BOOST TIP** Cinnamon can help improve insulin resistance and support proper ovarian function. Consume at least ½ teaspoon per day to improve insulin resistance.

PER SERVING Calories: 171; Carbohydrates: 0g; Glycemic Load: 0; Fiber: 0g; Protein: 34g; Sodium: 87mg; Fat: 4g

Fish Tacos with Root Vegetable Slaw

30-Minute, Dairy-Free, Inflammation Fighter

Serves 4 Fish tacos are an easy way to enjoy flaky fresh fish and an assortment of healthy vegetables in a neat and portable package. Haddock is a delightful fish choice because of its snowy mild-flavored flesh. It is an outstanding source of omega-3 fatty acids and protein as well as a good source of vitamin B_{12}, iron, and zinc. Haddock is also one of the fish flagged as low-mercury, which is important for women who have PCOS.

PREP: 15 minutes
COOK: 6 minutes

FOR THE SLAW

¼ head red cabbage, shredded

1 carrot, shredded

1 tablespoon freshly squeezed lemon juice

1 teaspoon raw honey

2 tablespoons chopped fresh cilantro leaves

FOR THE TACOS

1 tablespoon extra-virgin olive oil

4 (4-ounce) haddock fillets

4 (6-inch) sprouted tortillas

TO MAKE THE SLAW

In a medium bowl, toss together all the ingredients. Set aside.

TO MAKE THE TACOS

1. In a large skillet over medium-high heat, heat the olive oil.

2. Add the fillets and panfry for about 3 minutes per side, until cooked through and the fish flakes easily with a fork, turning once.

3. Arrange the tortillas on a clean work surface. Place 1 fish fillet in the middle of each. Spoon the slaw on the fish and fold the tortillas in half.

LOWER CALORIE TIP The tortillas add about 150 calories per serving, with 100 milligrams of sodium and 4 grams of fat. Replacing the tortillas with kale leaves reduces the calories by 120 and drops the sodium by 71 milligrams per serving. Kale also has 0 grams of fat and an abundance of nutrients.

PER SERVING Calories: 342; Carbohydrates: 32g; Glycemic Load: 5; Fiber: 8g; Protein: 30g; Sodium: 223mg; Fat: 10g

Seared Lemon Scallops

5-Ingredient, 30-Minute, Dairy-Free, Fertility Boost, Gluten-Free, Inflammation Fighter, Lower Calorie

Serves 4 Scallops have a mild, sweet flavor and a tender texture that is a lovely treat if you want a special-occasion dinner choice. Scallops are a superb source of vitamin B_{12}, a vitamin that can help prevent miscarriage, and iodine, a crucial component in hormone production in the thyroid gland. Scallops are low in calories and high in omega-3 fatty acids, phosphorous, protein, and choline. These nutrients support healthy fertility and fight inflammation, two important considerations for PCOS.

PREP: 10 minutes
COOK: 10 minutes

2 pounds sea scallops, cleaned and patted dry

Sea salt, for seasoning

Freshly ground black pepper, for seasoning

2 tablespoons extra-virgin olive oil

1 tablespoon minced garlic

Zest and juice of 1 lemon

1 teaspoon chopped fresh thyme leaves

1. Lightly season the scallops with salt and pepper on both sides.

2. In a large skillet over medium-high heat, heat the olive oil.

3. Add the garlic and sauté for about 2 minutes until softened.

4. Arrange the scallops in the skillet. Pan sear them for about 4 minutes per side, until they are just cooked through, turning once.

5. Remove the skillet from the heat and stir in the lemon zest and juice and the thyme.

FERTILITY BOOST TIP Citrus fruit is very high in potassium, folate, calcium, and vitamin C, which is an effective combination to regulate ovulation. Aim to enjoy at least one serving of citrus fruit, such as oranges, grapefruit, lemons, and tangerines, per day.

PER SERVING Calories: 260; Carbohydrates: 6g; Glycemic Load: 6; Fiber: 0g; Protein: 28g; Sodium: 385mg; Fat: 8g

Curried Seafood Soup

Dairy-Free, Gluten-Free, Inflammation Fighter, Lower Calorie

Serves 4 Imagine settling in after a long day with a bowl of fragrant, restorative soup studded with chunks of sweet shrimp, tender white fish, and earthy kale. Curry is an inspired flavoring that can be adjusted depending on your preference for heat. The combination of spices in curry, including turmeric, ginger, cumin, and cardamom, is great for fighting inflammation. Curry can also support heart and bone health and reduce the risk of cancer.

PREP: 10 minutes
COOK: 25 minutes

1 tablespoon extra-virgin olive oil

1 sweet onion, chopped

2 teaspoons grated fresh ginger

2 teaspoons minced garlic

8 cups low-sodium chicken broth

2 tablespoons red curry paste

3 celery stalks, chopped

2 carrots, chopped

1 pound haddock, cut into 1-inch chunks

½ pound chopped shrimp

1 cup chopped kale

1. In a large saucepan over medium-high heat, heat the olive oil.

2. Add the onion, ginger, and garlic and sauté for about 3 minutes, until softened.

3. Stir in the broth, curry paste, celery, and carrots. Bring the soup to a boil. Reduce the heat to low and simmer for 10 minutes.

4. Add the fish and shrimp and simmer for 10 minutes more.

5. Stir in the kale and simmer for 2 minutes.

INFLAMMATION FIGHTER TIP There is a generous amount of garlic in this recipe, and this allium is a powerful anti-oxidant, antibacterial, antiviral, and antifungal agent. The sulfur-containing compound allicin in garlic produces sulfenic acid when it breaks down in the body. Sulfenic acid can neutralize free radicals in the body with rapid response.

PER SERVING Calories: 242; Carbohydrates: 10g; Glycemic Load: 5; Fiber: 2g; Protein: 36g; Sodium: 245mg; Fat: 6g

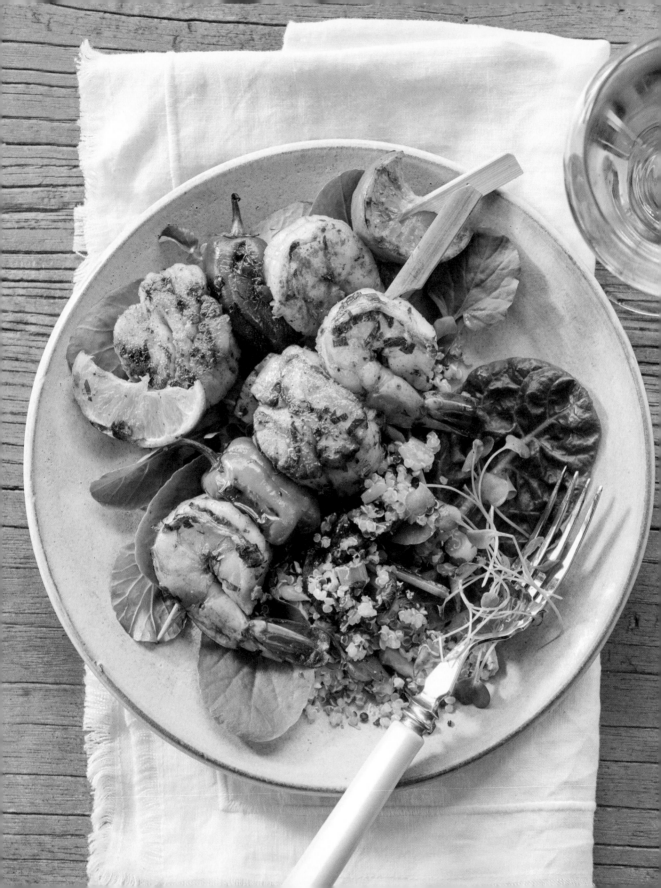

Roasted Shrimp with Peppers and Lime

Dairy-Free, Fertility Boost, Gluten-Free, Inflammation Fighter, Lower Calorie

Serves 4   Shrimp are a fabulous source of antioxidants, copper, selenium, and vitamin B_{12}. The most prevalent antioxidant in shrimp is astaxanthin, which is responsible for the pretty pink color of the flesh and is an effective anti-inflammatory agent. Vitamin B_{12} can reduce the risk of miscarriage by strengthening the endometrial lining and regulating estrogen levels. Deficiency of this vitamin has been linked to abnormal estrogen levels.

PREP: 15 minutes, plus 1 hour marinating time
COOK: 15 minutes

2 tablespoons extra-virgin olive oil

2 tablespoons freshly squeezed lemon juice

1 tablespoon chopped fresh basil leaves

2 teaspoons minced garlic

1 pound (16 to 20 count) shrimp, peeled and deveined

4 poblano peppers

2 limes, halved

Sea salt, for seasoning

Freshly ground black pepper, for seasoning

1. Preheat the oven to 450°F.

2. In a medium bowl, stir together the olive oil, lemon juice, basil, and garlic.

3. Stir in the shrimp and refrigerate for 1 hour to marinate.

4. Onto each of 4 skewers, thread the shrimp, 1 pepper, and 1 lime half. Place the skewers on a baking sheet and roast for about 15 minutes, turning once, until the shrimp are cooked through.

5. Season with salt and pepper, squeeze the lime half over each, and serve the skewers.

> **COOKING TIP** You can use any type of pepper, such as jalapeño or habanero, for these pretty skewers depending on your preference for heat. Poblanos are very mild so are great for people who want to experience spicy food without scorching heat.

PER SERVING Calories: 187; Carbohydrates: 3g; Glycemic Load: 2; Fiber: 0g; Protein: 23g; Sodium: 166mg; Fat: 9g

Haddock with Creamy Leeks

Dairy-Free, Fertility Boost, Gluten-Free

Serves 4 This dish is exquisite looking—creamy sauce with bright green leeks spooned over flaky, perfectly braised fish. Leeks are an allium—you should consume one serving of this type of vegetable every day. Leeks are high in vitamin K, manganese, copper, folate, and the flavonoid kaempferol. Folate is distributed throughout this plant, both in the white and green parts, so leeks are a wonderful pre-pregnancy and pregnancy food choice.

PREP: 10 minutes
COOK: 25 minutes

4 slices uncured bacon, diced

½ cup chopped sweet onion

1 teaspoon minced garlic

3 leeks, white and light green parts, cleaned and thinly sliced

½ cup low-sodium chicken broth

¼ cup coconut milk

4 (6-ounce) haddock fillets

1. In a large skillet over medium-high heat, sauté the bacon for about 5 minutes, until it is cooked through.

2. Stir in the onion and garlic. Sauté for about 3 minutes, until the vegetables soften.

3. Add the leeks and sauté for about 5 minutes, until tender.

4. Stir in the broth and coconut milk and bring to a simmer.

5. Add the haddock, cover, and cook for about 10 minutes, until the fish is just cooked through.

6. Serve the haddock topped with the leeks.

FERTILITY BOOST TIP Selenium is a powerful antioxidant that protects the ova from chromosomal damage that can cause miscarriage or birth defects. Haddock is very high in selenium—about 62 micrograms per 6-ounce portion, which is about 88 percent of the recommended daily amount for reproductive health.

PER SERVING Calories: 354; Carbohydrates: 12g; Glycemic Load: 4; Fiber: 2g; Protein: 36g; Sodium: 127mg; Fat: 16g

Steamed Sesame Trout with Bok Choy

30-Minute, Dairy-Free, Fertility Boost, Gluten-Free, Inflammation Fighter, Lower Calorie

Serves 4 Trout can be found in the fish section of most grocery stores; sometimes specialty grocery stores keep them in tanks so you can choose the one you want and have it cleaned for you. Trout is a freshwater fish so it is low in mercury. It is actually best to source farmed fish because the pools are protected from environmental contaminants. Trout is very high in inflammation-fighting omega-3 fatty acids and protein, which are crucial for good egg quality and increasing the likelihood of conception.

PREP: 10 minutes
COOK: 15 minutes

4 (5-ounce) trout fillets, patted dry

Sea salt, for seasoning

1 teaspoon sesame oil

2 teaspoons grated fresh ginger

1 teaspoon minced garlic

¼ cup water

4 cups shredded bok choy

1 tablespoon sesame seeds

1. Season the fish lightly with salt.

2. In a large skillet over medium-high heat, heat the sesame oil.

3. Add the ginger and garlic and sauté for about 3 minutes, until softened.

4. Add the water and bok choy and cover the skillet. Steam the bok choy for 5 minutes.

5. Add the fish. Cover the skillet and steam the fish for about 6 minutes, until it is just cooked through.

6. Serve topped with sesame seeds.

COOKING TIP If you have a steamer, use it instead of a skillet for this dish. Place the ginger, garlic, bok choy, and fish in the steamer. When tender and cooked through, drizzle with sesame oil, sprinkle with the sesame seeds, and serve.

PER SERVING Calories: 247; Carbohydrates: 3g; Glycemic Load: 1; Fiber: 1g; Protein: 31g; Sodium: 131mg; Fat: 11g

Sautéed Shrimp with Veggie Noodles

30-Minute, Dairy-Free, Fertility Boost, Gluten-Free, Inflammation Fighter, Lower Calorie

Serves 4 Vegetable noodles are a popular culinary application because they are versatile, low in calories, fat-free, and absolutely charming. Zucchini is one popular choice because it is flexible enough to spiralize easily and the flavor combines beautifully with many other ingredients. Zucchini contains powerful antioxidants, such as lutein and zeaxanthin. Leave the skin on because this part of the zucchini is very rich in antioxidants.

PREP: 15 minutes
COOK: 10 minutes

2 tablespoons extra-virgin olive oil

1 pound (16 to 20 count) shrimp, peeled and deveined

1 teaspoon minced garlic

¼ cup low-sodium chicken broth, or vegetable broth

Zest and juice of 1 lemon

1½ pounds zucchini, spiralized or julienned

Sea salt, for seasoning

Freshly ground black pepper, for seasoning

2 teaspoons chopped fresh oregano leaves

1. In a large skillet over medium-high heat, heat the olive oil.

2. Add the shrimp and garlic and sauté for about 5 minutes, until the shrimp are just cooked through.

3. Move the shrimp to the side of the skillet and stir in the broth and the lemon zest and juice. Bring the liquid to a simmer.

4. Stir in the zucchini. Simmer for 2 minutes.

5. Season with salt and pepper and serve garnished with oregano.

FERTILITY BOOST TIP Add ½ cup diced avocado per serving to top this fabulously fresh-looking dish. Avocado is a wonderful source of folate, vitamin K, and potassium. These nutrients can help regulate hormones and support the growth of a healthy fetus.

PER SERVING Calories: 215; Carbohydrates: 6g; Glycemic Load: 5; Fiber: 2g; Protein: 27g; Sodium: 171mg; Fat: 9g

Coconut-Breaded Tilapia

5-Ingredient, 30-Minute, Dairy-Free, Fertility Boost, Inflammation Fighter

Serves 4 Tilapia is a good PCOS protein choice because the fish don't accumulate damaging mercury due to their short life span. Tilapia is high in lean protein, omega-3 fatty acids, vitamins B_6 and B_{12}, and selenium. One 4-ounce serving contains more than 15 percent of the recommended daily amount of protein.

PREP: 10 minutes
COOK: 20 minutes

½ cup almond flour

2 large eggs, beaten

½ cup panko bread crumbs, toasted

½ cup unsweetened shredded coconut

4 (5-ounce) tilapia fillets, patted dry

1. Preheat the oven to 400°F.

2. At your workstation, line up 3 small bowls. In the first bowl, place the almond flour. In the second, place the beaten eggs. In the third, stir together the bread crumbs and coconut.

3. Dredge the fillets into the almond flour, dip into the eggs, and dredge in the coconut mixture until completely coated. Place the fillets on a baking sheet.

4. Bake the fish for about 20 minutes, until just cooked through.

FERTILITY BOOST TIP Replace the almond flour with an equal amount of ground flaxseed to increase the omega-3 fatty acids in the dish. Omega-3s can help decrease the risk of premature birth and miscarriage.

PER SERVING Calories: 309; Carbohydrates: 12g; Glycemic Load: 7; Fiber: 2g; Protein: 35g; Sodium: 212mg; Fat: 13g

Avocado Stuffed with Salmon Salad

30-Minute, Fertility Boost, Gluten-Free, Inflammation Fighter, Lower Calorie

Serves 4 The ingredients for this attractive dish are packed with healthy fats and other nutrients that support a PCOS diet. Avocado is a potent anti-inflammatory ingredient, rich in omega-3 fatty acids, manganese, selenium, vitamins C and E, and antioxidants such as lutein and beta-carotene. Yogurt is the source of beneficial bacteria and the good saturated fat required to support effective fertility.

PREP: 20 minutes
COOK: none

2 avocados, peeled, halved, and pitted

Juice of 1 lemon, divided

12 ounces cooked salmon

1 celery stalk, chopped

1 scallion, white and green parts, chopped

2 tablespoons plain low-fat yogurt

Sea salt, for seasoning

Freshly ground black pepper, for seasoning

1. Scoop out the hollow section of each avocado half and reserve the flesh for another recipe.

2. Rub the cut edges of the avocados with half the lemon juice and set them aside.

3. In a medium bowl, flake the fish with a fork.

4. Stir in the celery, scallion, yogurt, and remaining lemon juice. Season the salmon mixture with salt and pepper.

5. Scoop the salmon salad into the avocado halves and serve.

FERTILITY BOOST TIP Salmon is high in coenzyme Q-10 (CoQ10), with about 2.3 milligrams per 3-ounce serving. CoQ10 can increase ova (egg) health and, as an antioxidant, protect DNA from damage. Enjoy this nutrition-packed fish at least once a week.

PER SERVING Calories: 282; Carbohydrates: 7g; Glycemic Load: 2; Fiber: 5g; Protein: 20g; Sodium: 61mg; Fat: 20g

Baked Salmon with Peach Salsa

30-Minute, Dairy-Free, Fertility Boost, Gluten-Free, Inflammation Fighter

Serves 4 If you want a taste of summer, whip up this dish in the winter months for a festive lift of spirits. The colors and freshness of the salsa is glorious and indicates the presence of antioxidants such as beta-carotene and lycopene. Salmon is a known source of inflammation busting omega-3 fatty acids and is high the protein that is vital to fertility.

PREP: 15 minutes
COOK: 15 minutes

FOR THE SALSA

1 peach, chopped

1 scallion, white and green parts, chopped

½ red bell pepper, chopped

½ cup chopped cucumber

Juice of ½ lime

Pinch red pepper flakes

FOR THE FISH

4 (5-ounce) skinless salmon filets

¼ teaspoon sea salt

¼ teaspoon freshly ground black pepper

1 tablespoon extra-virgin olive oil

FOR THE SALSA

In a small bowl, stir together the peach, scallion, red bell pepper, cucumber, lime juice, and red pepper flakes. Set aside.

FOR THE FISH

1. Preheat the oven to 400°F. Line a small baking sheet with aluminum foil and set aside.

2. Rub the sea salt and black pepper onto both sides of the fish and place them on the prepared sheet.

3. Drizzle the fish with olive oil.

4. Bake for about 15 minutes, until the salmon flakes easily.

5. Serve with the salsa.

> **INGREDIENT TIP** Wild-caught salmon is considered to be healthy, but the best choice if it suits your budget is wild-caught Alaskan salmon because it is lowest in environmental contaminants. This fish is also one of the more sustainable choices.

PER SERVING Calories: 329; Carbohydrates: 5g; Glycemic Load: 1; Fiber: 1g; Protein: 212g; Sodium: 28mg; Fat: 21g

7

Poultry and Meat Entrées

Easy Chicken Chili

30-Minute, Dairy-Free, Gluten-Free, Fertility Boost, Inflammation Fighter, Lower Calorie

Serves 4 Chicken breast is a popular ingredient in many diets meant to support good health, which makes sense because skinless chicken breasts are very low in fat and high in protein. Chicken is also rich in vitamins B_3, B_5, and B_6, selenium, potassium, and amino acids. Vitamins B_3 and B_5 help convert carbohydrates, like the navy beans, and fats, like the olive oil, to energy. Vitamin B_6 is essential for hormone balance, converting glycogen to glucose, and is required for zinc absorption in the intestines.

PREP: 10 minutes
COOK: 20 minutes

1 tablespoon extra-virgin olive oil

½ sweet onion, chopped

2 teaspoons grated fresh ginger

1 teaspoon minced garlic

2 (5-ounce) cooked boneless skinless chicken breasts, shredded

2 cups canned sodium-free navy beans, drained and rinsed

1 (14.5-ounce) can sodium-free diced tomatoes, undrained

1½ tablespoons chili powder

1 teaspoon ground cumin

Pinch cayenne pepper

1. In a large saucepan over medium-high heat, heat the olive oil.

2. Add the onion, ginger, and garlic and sauté for about 3 minutes, until softened.

3. Stir in the chicken, navy beans, tomatoes, chili powder, cumin, and cayenne. Bring the chili to a boil, reduce the heat to low, and simmer for 15 minutes.

FERTILITY BOOST TIP Legumes, such as the navy beans in this chili, are a spectacular source of plant protein. Eating plant protein can reduce the risk of having trouble conceiving. Include at least 1 serving of legumes or beans per day to reap the benefits of lots of protein, fiber, folate, and iron.

PER SERVING Calories: 295; Carbohydrates: 29g; Glycemic Load: 8; Fiber: 11g; Protein: 30g; Sodium: 75mg; Fat: 7g

Pork Fajita Roll-Ups

Dairy-Free, Fertility Boost, Gluten-Free, Inflammation Fighter, Lower Calorie

Serves 4 Pork is consumed more than any other red meat in the world and is a very healthy choice—high in protein, thiamine, vitamins B_6 and B_{12}, zinc, and iron. Including pork in your diet several times a week can reduce the risk of a vitamin B_6 deficiency, which has been linked to irregular menstruation and improper egg production. The colorful bell peppers add an anti-inflammatory component because they are loaded with antioxidants and vitamin C.

PREP: 10 minutes, plus 1 hour marinating time
COOK: 25 minutes

1 tablespoon extra-virgin olive oil

Zest and juice of 1 lime

1 teaspoon minced garlic

1 teaspoon dried oregano

½ teaspoon ground cumin

4 (4-ounce) pork chops, cut horizontally through the middle to within ½ inch of cutting all the way through

1 red bell pepper, sliced

1 yellow bell pepper, sliced

1 red onion, thinly sliced

1. In a medium bowl, whisk the olive oil, lime zest and juice, garlic, oregano, and cumin.

2. On your work surface, spread the pork chops open and pound them to ¼-inch thickness. Add them to the marinade, cover the bowl, and refrigerate for 1 hour.

3. Preheat the oven to 400°F.

4. Remove the pork chops from the marinade and spread them open again on your work surface.

5. Divide the bell pepper slices and onion among the chops and roll them up. Secure the rolls with toothpicks placed in the middle and place them seam-side down in a baking dish.

6. Bake for about 25 minutes, until the pork is cooked through.

INGREDIENT TIP Pork tenderloins can be used instead of pork chops; just cut them and pound them flat like the chops. Pork tenderloins should also be trimmed of silverskin and extra fat.

PER SERVING Calories: 293; Carbohydrates: 6g; Glycemic Load: 2; Fiber: 2g; Protein: 22g; Sodium: 50mg; Fat: 17g

Tarragon Turkey with Navy Beans

Dairy-Free, Fertility Boost, Gluten-Free, Inflammation Fighter

Serves 4 Tarragon is an extremely popular herb in Mediterranean and French cuisines, and its sweet anise flavor enhances the taste of the turkey and navy beans in this dish. Tarragon has one of the highest antioxidant profiles of any herb and is an excellent source of phytonutrients and polyphenolic compounds that help lower blood sugar levels. Tarragon is also an excellent source of vitamins A, B complex, and C, as well as calcium and iron.

PREP: 10 minutes
COOK: 25 minutes

16 ounces boneless skinless turkey breast, cut into 2-inch chunks

Sea salt, for seasoning

Freshly ground black pepper, for seasoning

1 tablespoon extra-virgin olive oil, divided

2 celery stalks, sliced

1 sweet onion, cut into eighths

1 teaspoon minced garlic

½ cup low-sodium chicken broth

1 (14-ounce) can sodium-free navy beans, drained and rinsed

1 tablespoon chopped fresh tarragon leaves

1. Lightly season the turkey with salt and pepper.

2. In a large skillet over medium-high heat, heat the olive oil.

3. Add the turkey and brown for 5 minutes, turning once halfway through. Transfer the turkey to a plate.

4. Return the skillet to the heat and add the celery, onion, and garlic. Sauté for 3 minutes, breaking up the onion.

5. Stir in the chicken broth and return the turkey to the skillet. Bring the mixture to a boil. Reduce the heat to low and simmer for about 10 minutes, until the turkey is cooked through.

6. Stir in the navy beans and tarragon and simmer for 5 minutes.

FERTILITY BOOST TIP Turkey is a fabulous source of vitamin B_6—about 54 percent of the recommended daily amount is in each serving of this dish. Vitamin B_6 can improve the quality of the body's eggs as well as regulate and increase the luteal phase of the menstrual cycle. Consider using turkey in your recipes instead of other proteins.

PER SERVING Calories: 303; Carbohydrates: 28g; Glycemic Load: 8; Fiber: 11g; Protein: 36g; Sodium: 84mg; Fat: 5g

Pork Vegetable Confetti Meatballs

5-Ingredient, 30-Minute, Dairy-Free, Gluten-Free, Inflammation Fighter

Serves 4 Meatballs are a handy meal because they can be used in so many ways—plain, in a savory sauce, tucked into a sprouted pita pocket, or added to a casserole. The vegetables in these lean meatballs add color, bulk, and a healthy amount of fiber and antioxidants.

PREP: 10 minutes
COOK: 15 minutes

1 pound ground pork

¼ cup shredded carrot

1 tablespoon chopped fresh basil leaves

1 teaspoon minced garlic

Dash sea salt

Dash freshly ground black pepper

1 tablespoon extra-virgin olive oil

1. In a large bowl, thoroughly mix the pork, carrot, basil, garlic, salt, and pepper. Form the pork mixture into 12 meatballs.

2. In a large skillet over medium-high heat, heat the olive oil.

3. Add the meatballs and brown on all sides for about 15 minutes, or until they are cooked through.

4. Serve warm or cold.

> **LOWER CALORIE TIP** Baking these tender meatballs instead of panfrying them can reduce the calories by about 30 and eliminate 3 grams of fat per serving. Arrange the meatballs on a rimmed baking sheet and bake in a 400°F for 20 to 25 minutes, turning once.

PER SERVING (3 meatballs) Calories: 334; Carbohydrates: 2g; Glycemic Load: 1; Fiber: 1g; Protein: 19g; Sodium: 81mg; Fat: 25g

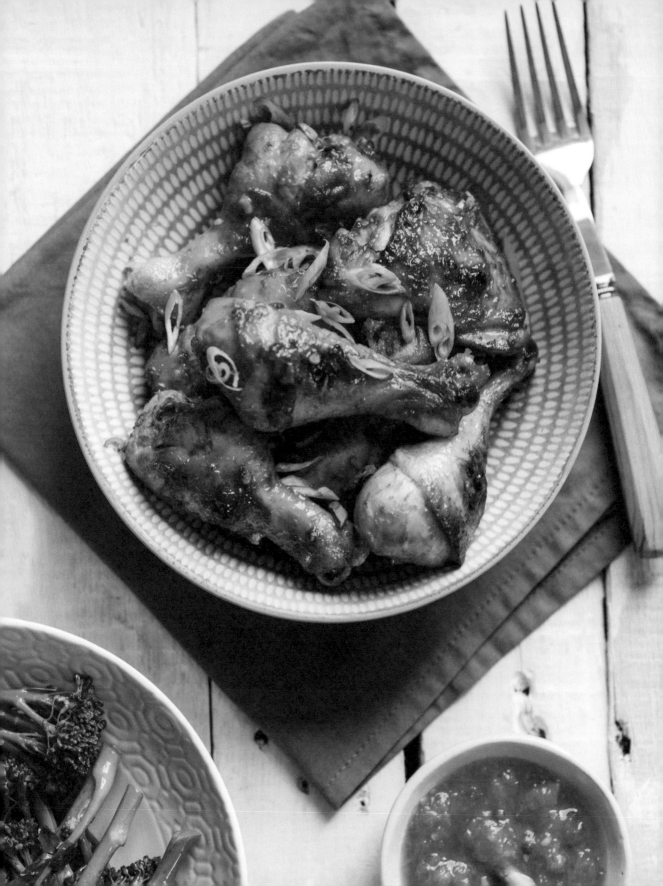

Roasted Chicken with Asian Glaze

Dairy-Free, Fertility Boost, Gluten-Free, Inflammation Fighter

Serves 4 The sauce for this chicken is delectable—and flavored with sesame and rich garlic undertones. You might want to toss it with pasta or braise other proteins, such as halibut or pork, in it. Garlic is well-known for its anti-inflammatory properties, but it can also boost fertility because it is high in selenium. Selenium can help prevent miscarriage and is important for egg production.

PREP: 10 minutes, plus 1 hour marinating time
COOK: 30 minutes

¼ cup apple cider vinegar

2 tablespoons sesame sauce

2 tablespoons coconut aminos

1 tablespoon raw honey

1 teaspoon minced garlic

½ teaspoon chili paste

8 chicken pieces, drumsticks and thighs

1 scallion, green part only, thinly sliced on a bias

1. In a large bowl, stir together the vinegar, sesame sauce, coconut aminos, honey, garlic, and chili paste until well blended.

2. Add the chicken and toss to coat. Refrigerate the chicken for 1 hour to marinate, turning once.

3. Preheat the oven to 350°F.

4. Arrange the chicken on a baking sheet and roast for about 30 minutes, until cooked through and lightly caramelized.

5. Serve topped with the scallion.

> **FERTILITY BOOST TIP** Top this dish with a couple of table-spoons of plain Greek yogurt because it is high in vitamin D, calcium, and protein. Vitamin D helps the ovaries' follicles mature and boosts your immune system.

PER SERVING Calories: 319; Carbohydrates: 5g; Glycemic Load: 3; Fiber: 0g; Protein: 28g; Sodium: 176mg; Fat: 16g

Spanish Chicken

Dairy-Free, Fertility Boost, Gluten-Free, Inflammation Fighter, Lower Calorie

Serves 4 Simple is sometimes exactly what you are looking for when you do not want to slave over the stove. This is meal has very few ingredients but they make an impact flavor-wise, boost fertility, and improve general health. Tomatoes and bell peppers are antioxidant, and rich in vitamin C and fiber. These nutrients improve the chances of conceiving and create an ideal environment for fetal development.

PREP: 10 minutes
COOK: 30 minutes

1 tablespoon coconut oil

4 (5-ounce) skinless, boneless chicken breast, cut into 2-inch chunks

1 sweet onion, chopped

½ jalapeño pepper, finely chopped

1 tablespoon minced garlic

1½ tablespoons smoked paprika

1 teaspoon ground ginger

2 red bell peppers, diced

1 (14.5-ounce) can sodium-free diced tomatoes, undrained

1 cup low-sodium chicken broth

1. In a large skillet over medium-high heat, heat the coconut oil. Add the chicken and brown for 5 minutes.

2. Transfer the chicken to a plate.

3. Return the skillet to the heat and add the onion, jalapeño pepper, garlic, paprika, and ginger. Sauté for 3 minutes, until translucent.

4. Stir in the red peppers, tomatoes, chicken broth and return the chicken to the skillet.

5. Bring the mixture to a boil.

6. Reduce the heat to low and simmer for about 20 minutes, until the chicken is cooked through.

COOKING TIP If you do not like using canned tomatoes, 3 large fresh tomatoes can be chopped and thrown in the sauce. Look for ripe produce with firm unblemished skin and a strong tomato scent.

PER SERVING   Calories: 231; Carbohydrates: 11g; Glycemic Load: 3; Fiber: 3g; Protein: 34g; Sodium: 105mg; Fat: 6g

Pork Chops with Mediterranean Vegetables

Dairy-Free, Fertility Boost, Gluten-Free, Inflammation Fighter, Lower Calorie

Serves 4 The Mediterranean diet is considered one of the healthiest in the world—featuring olive oil, garlic, heaps of nutritious vegetables, and lean proteins. This entire recipe contains all the elements of this fantastic diet. The oregano is rich in vitamin K, manganese, iron, calcium, and fiber. Oregano is also packed with phytonutrients, including thymol and rosmarinic acid, and this humble little herb, by volume, has more antioxidant activity than many other high-antioxidant foods, such as apples, blueberries, and citrus fruits.

PREP: 10 minutes
COOK: 22 minutes

16 ounces boneless pork chops

Sea salt, for seasoning

Freshly ground black pepper, for seasoning

1 tablespoon extra-virgin olive oil

½ red onion, thinly sliced

2 teaspoons minced garlic

1 zucchini, shredded

1 yellow summer squash, shredded

1 cup halved grape tomatoes

2 teaspoons fresh oregano leaves

¼ cup sliced black olives

1. Season the pork chops with salt and pepper and thinly slice the meat.

2. In a large skillet over medium-high heat, heat the olive oil.

3. Add the pork and sauté for about 10 minutes until just cooked through. Transfer the pork to a plate.

4. Return the skillet to the heat, add the onion and garlic, and sauté for 2 minutes.

5. Stir in the zucchini, squash, tomatoes, and oregano. Sauté for about 10 minutes until heated through.

6. Return the pork to the skillet and stir to combine.

7. Serve topped with the olives.

INGREDIENT TIP Oregano is a popular herb in Mediterranean cooking and it is also one of the easiest herbs to grow yourself. Cultivate oregano in window boxes or pots, year-round, so you always have a handy, healthy flavor boost nearby.

PER SERVING Calories: 296; Carbohydrates: 4g; Glycemic Load: 1; Fiber: 1g; Protein: 23g; Sodium: 235mg; Fat: 19g

Baked Parsley Lamb

5-Ingredient, 30-Minute, Dairy-Free, Fertility Boost, Gluten-Free

Serves 4 Parsley is much more than a simple garnish to be tossed aside while you eat; it is a powerhouse of important nutrients. Parsley has a stellar quantity of vitamin K: more than 500 percent of the recommended amount in as little as ½ cup. Parsley is also high in vitamins A and C as well as folate, iron, and copper, so it should be a regular ingredient in your PCOS-friendly meals. These nutrients support fertility, and its plentiful antioxidants, such as lutein, fight inflammation.

PREP: 10 minutes
COOK: 15 minutes

2 tablespoons extra-virgin olive oil, divided

¼ cup fresh parsley sprigs

1 tablespoon chopped fresh thyme leaves

1 teaspoon minced garlic

Pinch sea salt

Pinch freshly ground black pepper

4 (5-ounce) lamb chops

1. Preheat the oven to 400°F.

2. In a blender, combine 4 teaspoons olive oil, the parsley, thyme, garlic, salt, and pepper. Pulse until a thick paste forms.

3. In a large skillet over medium-high heat, heat the remaining 2 teaspoons olive oil.

4. Add the lamb chops. Pan sear on all sides for about 5 minutes total and place them in a baking dish.

5. Spread the parsley mixture over the chops.

6. Bake the chops for about 10 minutes for medium, or until your desired doneness.

FERTILITY BOOST TIP Lamb is rich in vitamin B_{12} (cobalamin)—about 54 percent of the recommended daily amount per 5-ounce serving. B_{12} can increase the endometrial lining when the egg is fertilized, which can reduce the risk of miscarriage. A deficiency of this vitamin can create irregular or absent ovulation, so it is important to meet the recommended daily amount whenever possible.

PER SERVING Calories: 353; Carbohydrates: 0g; Glycemic Load: 0; Fiber: 0g; Protein: 26g; Sodium: 97mg; Fat: 25g

Lamb-Ginger Burgers

Dairy-Free, Inflammation Fighter

Serves 4 Sometimes, quality ingredients are hard to find or are more expensive, so justifying the purchase price is difficult. In the case of lamb, however, grass-fed is worth the extra money. Grass-fed lamb has higher levels of omega-3 fatty acids—about 25 percent more than factory-raised animals. Grass-fed lamb has more than 50 percent more alpha-linolenic acid (ALA), a building block of omega-3 fatty acids. Lamb's overall fat content is also reduced when the animals are grass fed, by a minimum of 15 percent.

PREP: 10 minutes, plus
10 minutes cooling time
COOK: 13 minutes

1 tablespoon extra-virgin olive oil, divided

½ sweet onion, chopped

2 teaspoons grated fresh ginger

1 teaspoon minced garlic

1 pound ground lamb

2 tablespoons panko bread crumbs

½ teaspoon chopped fresh thyme leaves

Dash sea salt

Dash freshly ground black pepper

1. In a small skillet over medium-high heat, heat 1 teaspoon olive oil.

2. Add the onion, ginger, and garlic and sauté for about 3 minutes, until softened. Transfer the onion mixture to a medium bowl and let it cool for 10 minutes.

3. To the bowl, add the lamb, bread crumbs, thyme, salt, and pepper. Mix until well combined. Divide the lamb mixture into 4 equal portions and form each into a ½-inch-thick patty.

4. In a large skillet over medium-high heat, heat the remaining 2 teaspoons olive oil.

5. Add the burgers and panfry for about 5 minutes per side until lightly browned for medium-well, or until your desired doneness. Serve immediately.

LOWER CALORIE TIP This recipe assumes you will use ground lamb available from most supermarket meat counters. Sourcing a good butcher, however, who can grind specific cuts of meat, can cut fat and calories. Ground leg of lamb, trimmed, can cut 100 calories and 9 grams of fat from these burgers as well as increase the protein by 2 grams per serving.

PER SERVING Calories: 379; Carbohydrates: 6g; Glycemic Load: 4; Fiber: 0g; Protein: 20g; Sodium: 130mg; Fat: 24g

Lamb Souvlaki

5-Ingredient, Dairy-Free, Fertility Boost, Gluten-Free, Inflammation Fighter, Lower Calorie

Serves 4 Lamb is a popular protein choice in many places in the world and is a fantastic source of omega-3 fatty acids, protein, and vitamin B$_{12}$. This combination can help prevent miscarriage and support healthy egg production. Include at least three lean protein servings per day, which should be about 15 percent to 20 percent of your total daily calories.

PREP: 15 minutes, plus 1 hour marinating time
COOK: 10 minutes

2 tablespoons freshly squeezed lemon juice

1 tablespoon extra-virgin olive oil

1 tablespoon chopped fresh oregano leaves

1 teaspoon ground cumin

¼ teaspoon freshly ground black pepper

⅛ teaspoon sea salt

1 pound lamb shoulder, cut into 1-inch chunks

1. In a medium bowl, whisk the lemon juice, olive oil, oregano, cumin, pepper, and salt.

2. Add the lamb to the bowl and stir to coat. Refrigerate the lamb, covered, for 1 hour to marinate.

3. Preheat the oven to broil.

4. Thread the lamb chunks onto 4 skewers. Place the skewers on a baking sheet and broil for about 10 minutes for medium, turning at least once, until your desired doneness.

FERTILITY BOOST TIP Add 1-inch chunks of yam to your lamb skewers because this sweet vegetable is thought to stimulate ovulation. Yams contain phytoestrogens and progesterone-like properties, which can help balance estrogen and progesterone in the body.

PER SERVING Calories: 263; Carbohydrates: 0g; Glycemic Load: 0; Fiber: 0g; Protein: 21g; Sodium: 78mg; Fat: 19g

Steak Diane Sauté

30-Minute, Dairy-Free, Fertility Boost, Gluten-Free, Inflammation Fighter, Lower Calorie

Serves 4 Zinc is crucial for cell division and balancing estrogen and progesterone levels. A deficiency of this mineral has been linked to miscarriage in the early stages of pregnancy. Beef is an excellent source of zinc and can be included weekly in a fertility-friendly diet. Look for grass-fed beef because it has double the carotenoids, beta-carotene, and lutein as conventionally farmed beef.

PREP: 5 minutes
COOK: 25 minutes

1 pound beef rump steak, trimmed and thinly sliced

Sea salt, for seasoning

Freshly ground black pepper, for seasoning

1 tablespoon extra-virgin olive oil, divided

4 ounces button mushrooms, sliced

¼ cup chopped sweet onion

1 teaspoon minced garlic

½ cup low-sodium beef broth

1 tablespoon Dijon mustard

¼ cup coconut cream

1 tablespoon chopped fresh parsley leaves

1. Lightly season the beef with salt and pepper.

2. Preheat a large skillet over medium-high heat and add 1 teaspoon olive oil.

3. Add the beef and sauté for about 10 minutes until just cooked through. With a slotted spoon, transfer the beef to a plate.

4. Return the skillet to the heat and add the remaining 2 teaspoons olive oil, mushrooms, onion, and garlic. Sauté for about 5 minutes, until tender.

5. Stir in the broth and mustard. Simmer for 10 minutes.

6. Stir in the coconut cream. Season the sauce with salt and pepper.

7. Return the beef to the skillet. Spoon the sauce over and top with parsley.

COOKING TIP You can buy precut beef, but purchasing an entire roast and trimming it yourself is less expensive. Look for beef with a little marbling because it will keep the meat tender in the limited cooking time.

PER SERVING Calories: 278; Carbohydrates: 3g; Glycemic Load: 1; Fiber: 1g; Protein: 25g; Sodium: 103mg; Fat: 18g

8

Drinks and Desserts

Creamy Kiwi Cucumber Smoothie

5-Ingredient, 30-Minute, Gluten-Free, Inflammation Fighter, Lower Calorie

Serves 2 Kiwi is a charming fruit—small, bright green or yellow, with tiny seeds. Kiwi is high in phytonutrients, vitamins C, E, and K, and fiber. The fiber in kiwi can help reduce blood sugar levels and lower cholesterol. This pale green smoothie counts as two vegetable servings, two fruit servings, and one dairy serving toward a balanced daily total. Sip and savor its goodness.

PREP: 10 minutes
COOK: none

1 English cucumber, chopped

2 kiwis, peeled and cut into chunks

½ cup plain low-fat yogurt

1 teaspoon freshly squeezed lemon juice

1 teaspoon chopped fresh mint leaves

In a blender, combine all the ingredients. Blend until smooth.

INFLAMMATION FIGHTER TIP Maintaining a healthy gut is crucial for fighting inflammation. Plain yogurt is one of the most accessible sources of live probiotics, which recolonize the gut with beneficial microbes. Increase the yogurt to 1 cup to double the positive impact of this creamy smoothie.

PER SERVING Calories: 104; Carbohydrates: 21g; Glycemic Load: 6; Fiber: 3g; Protein: 5g; Sodium: 44mg; Fat: 1g

Almond-Oatmeal Smoothie

5-Ingredient, 30-Minute, Dairy-Free, Fertility Boost, Inflammation Fighter, Lower Calorie

Serves 2 Sometimes smoothies are delicious but not very filling, so they are more a snack than a breakfast choice. This smoothie contains several sources of fiber—oats, apple, and chia seeds—and will keep you satisfied for hours, with no sugar spikes or cravings. Apples are one of the most nutritious foods on the planet and they contain small amounts of almost every nutrient. Apples are also incredibly high in antioxidants that help repair the effects of free radicals.

PREP: 5 minutes
COOK: none

1 cup unsweetened almond milk

1 apple, cored and cut into chunks

¼ cup rolled oats

1 tablespoon chia seeds

½ teaspoon pure vanilla extract

Pinch ground cinnamon

3 ice cubes

1. In a blender, combine the almond milk, apple, oats, chia seeds, vanilla, and cinnamon. Blend until smooth.

2. Add the ice and blend again until smooth and thick.

INFLAMMATION FIGHTER TIP The raw oats in this sweet smoothie pass through the gut undigested, which means they feed the friendly bacteria and boost inflammation-fighting fatty acids. Butyrate, one of these fatty acids, reduces insulin resistance while fighting inflammation. You can increase the amount of oats in the smoothie by a couple of tablespoons or include this breakfast choice more than once a week in your menu rotation.

PER SERVING Calories: 174; Carbohydrates: 30g; Glycemic Load: 8; Fiber: 6g; Protein: 5g; Sodium: 72mg; Fat: 4g

Peach Chia Smoothie

5-Ingredient, 30-Minute, Dairy Free, Gluten Free, Inflammation Fighter

Serves 2 Peaches are a high antioxidant fruit with marvelous health benefits and an absolutely fabulous taste. Stone fruit have an interesting combination of nutrients that can help reduce the risk of metabolic syndrome, diabetes, weight gain, and inflammation. Peaches contain antioxidants that can suppress the release of histamines in the blood that can cause inflammation and allergic reaction.

PREP: 5 minutes
COOK: none

1 cup unsweetened coconut milk

1 cup water

1 peach, pitted and chopped

3 tablespoons chia seeds

½ teaspoons ground nutmeg

Pinch ground allspice

4 ice cubes

1. In a blender, combine all the ingredients except the ice. Blend until smooth.

2. Add the ice and blend.

LOWER CALORIE TIP The calories in this creamy smoothie are not high if you intend on drinking it for breakfast. If you want lower numbers in calories and fat grams for a snack, you should swap out the coconut milk for unsweetened almond milk.

PER SERVING Calories: 385; Carbohydrates: 22g; Glycemic Load: 5; Fiber: 12g; Protein:7 g; Sodium: 20mg; Fat: 33g

Honeyed Carrot Mousse

Dairy-Free, Fertility Boost, Gluten-Free, Inflammation Fighter, Lower Calorie

---

Serves 4   If you avoid gelatin, you might be surprised at how easy this ingredient is to use. If you are a vegan or vegetarian, you'll want to use agar instead, because gelatin is made from animal collagen. Gelatin is a spectacular source of protein, and is low-calorie, fat-free, and sodium-free. This ingredient is currently being studied as a possible anti-inflammatory agent.

PREP: 10 minutes,
plus 1 hour chilling time
COOK: none

¼ cup unsweetened
almond milk

1 tablespoon
unflavored gelatin

2 cups mashed
cooked carrots

1 avocado, peeled, pitted,
and quartered

1 tablespoon raw honey

½ teaspoon ground
cinnamon

Pinch ground cloves

1. In a small bowl, add the almond milk. Sprinkle the gelatin evenly over the almond milk and let it sit for 10 minutes.

2. In a blender, combine the carrots, avocado, honey, cinnamon, and cloves. Process until silky smooth.

3. Spoon the mousse into a container and stir in the gelatin mixture. Cover the container and refrigerate for 1 hour to set.

4. Keep refrigerated in a sealed container for up to 2 days.

FERTILITY BOOST TIP Avocados contain several nutrients that support a healthy reproductive system, such as vitamin E to improve the endometrial lining and folate to reduce the risk of birth defects such as spina bifida. One avocado contains about 40 percent of the recommended daily amount of vitamin E and 60 percent of the required amount of folate.

PER SERVING Calories: 108; Carbohydrates: 14g; Glycemic Load: 5; Fiber: 4g; Protein: 3g; Sodium: 59mg; Fat: 6g

Coconut Almond Truffles

5-Ingedient, Dairy-Free, Gluten-Free, Inflammation Fighter, Lower Calorie

Makes 12 truffles Almond butter is rich, toasty, and a splendid alternative to peanut butter if allergies are an issue. This nut butter is a wonderful source of protein, folate, and calcium, and is low in saturated fat. Consuming almond butter can positively affect insulin resistance and stop cravings, so it is perfect for PCOS diets. The coconut and raw honey ensure these truffles are an inflammation-fighting snack as well as delicious.

PREP: 15 minutes, plus 1 hour chilling time
COOK: none

1 cup almond butter

1½ cups toasted unsweetened shredded coconut, divided

2 tablespoons raw honey

¼ teaspoon ground nutmeg

1. In a medium bowl, stir together the almond butter, 1 cup coconut, the honey, and nutmeg until well combined. Refrigerate the mixture for 1 hour, or until firm enough to roll.

2. Roll the mixture into 12 balls, and roll the balls in the remaining ½ cup coconut.

3. Refrigerate the coconut truffles in a sealed container for up to 1 week.

COOKING TIP Toasting coconut is extremely simple, especially unsweetened shreds, which do not burn as easily as products with added sugar. Spread the coconut on a baking sheet and toast in a 300°F oven, stirring occasionally, until the coconut is fragrant and golden brown.

PER SERVING (1 truffle) Calories: 189; Carbohydrates: 9g; Glycemic Load: 2; Fiber: 2g; Protein: 4g; Sodium: 5mg; Fat: 17g

Hazelnut Rice Pudding

5-Ingredient, Dairy-Free, Gluten-Free, Fertility Boost, Inflammation Fighter, Lower Calorie

Serves 4 Rice pudding is no longer that humble dessert served only in diners or home kitchens; it is on many fine-dining restaurant menus because rice combines beautifully with most ingredients. No matter where you enjoy it, it's sure to make you feel at home. Hazelnuts make a lovely topping—crunchy and sweet with many nutritional benefits—and support fertility with marvelous levels of folate, vitamin E, fiber, and monounsaturated fatty acids like oleic acid and linoleic acid. Look for unshelled raw nuts to avoid added preservatives.

PREP: 5 minutes
COOK: 30 minutes

1 cup unsweetened almond milk

¼ cup brown rice

2 tablespoons raw honey

2 teaspoons lemon zest

1 teaspoon pure vanilla extract

½ cup chopped hazelnuts

1. In a medium saucepot over medium heat, stir together the almond milk, brown rice, honey, lemon zest, and vanilla.

2. Bring to a boil, stirring occasionally. Reduce the heat to low and simmer for about 30 minutes, partially covered, stirring often, until the rice is tender.

3. Serve the pudding garnished with hazelnuts.

INGREDIENT TIP Make your own almond milk: Combine blanched almonds and water in a food processor (about 1 cup almonds and 4 cups water) and process until completely blended. Pass the liquid through a fine-mesh sieve or cheesecloth and refrigerate the milk in a sealed container for up to 1 week.

PER SERVING Calories: 179; Carbohydrates: 22g; Glycemic Load: 10; Fiber: 2g; Protein: 3g; Sodium: 36mg; Fat: 10g

Ruby Red Grapefruit Smoothie

5-Ingredient, 30-Minute, Fertility Boost, Gluten-Free, Inflammation Fighter, Lower Calorie

Serves 2 The ingredients in this pretty pale-pink smoothie are an ideal mix of PCOS-friendly choices. Grapefruit, strawberries, and spinach are high in fiber. Spinach is a stellar source of folic acid and iron, which support both conception and the development of the fetus. Yogurt is a healthy fat, high in protein, and contains healthy probiotic bacteria that promote gut health to reduce overall inflammation.

PREP: 10 minutes
COOK: none

1 ruby red grapefruit, peeled, pith removed

1 cup frozen strawberries

½ cup fresh spinach

½ cup water

¼ cup plain low-fat yogurt

In a blender, combine all the ingredients. Blend until smooth.

INFLAMMATION FIGHTER TIP Spinach is very high in vitamins C, E, and K as well as carotenoids, which all fight inflammation in the body. The form of vitamin E in spinach, alpha-tocopherol, is particularly effective for protecting the cardiovascular system. Eat at least 1 cup of spinach several times a week as a part of your meals.

PER SERVING Calories: 192; Carbohydrates: 41g; Glycemic Load: 12; Fiber: 7g; Protein: 3g; Sodium: 21mg; Fat: 1g

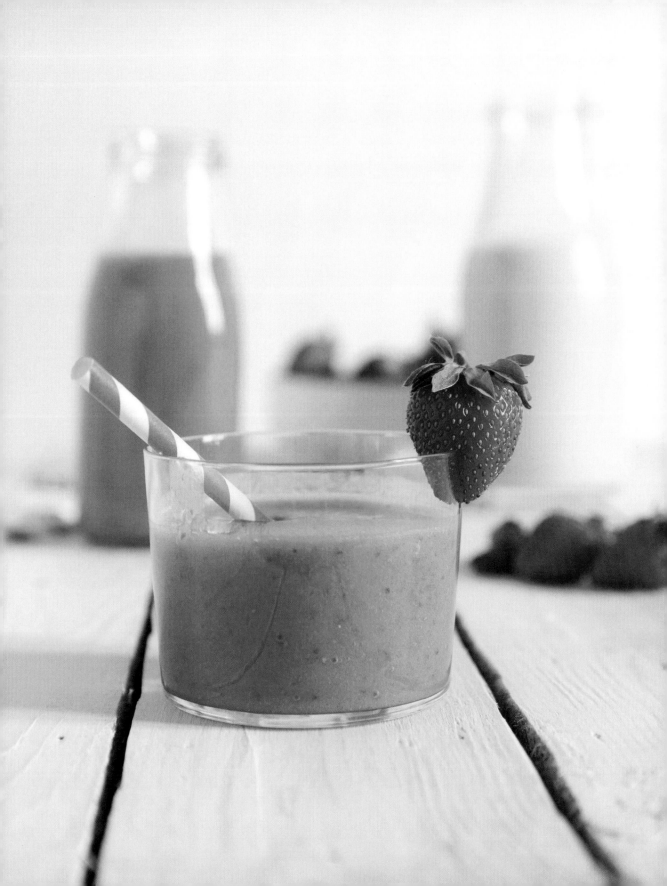

Pear-Anise Sorbet

5-Ingredient, Dairy-Free, Gluten-Free, Inflammation Fighter, Lower Calorie

Makes 2 cups Star anise is one of the prettiest spices because it looks like tiny reddish-brown stars. Star anise has a sweet, distinctly licorice-like flavor that is lovely with pears and a hint of honey. It contains several chemical compounds that are potent antioxidants, and this spice is also high in vitamins A, B, and C, calcium, iron, copper, potassium, manganese, and zinc. A treat for the senses, the body, and the spirit.

PREP: 10 minutes, plus 5 hours chilling time
COOK: 10 minutes

4 pears, peeled, cored, and cut into chunks

½ cup water

1 tablespoon raw honey

3 star anise

1. In a medium pot over medium-low heat, combine all the ingredients. Bring the mixture to a boil. Boil for 10 minutes and remove the pot from the heat. Let the mixture cool.

2. Remove and discard the star anise. Transfer the pear mixture to a blender and pulse until smooth. Pour the pear mixture into a metal baking dish and place the dish in the freezer.

3. Periodically, with a fork, scrape the edges as the mixture freezes. Repeat this process until the mixture resembles fine snow, about 5 hours total.

INFLAMMATION FIGHTER TIP Add 1 cup fresh blueberries to this frozen treat because this delectable blue fruit is packed with antioxidants and phytonutrients—in particular, a flavonoid family called anthocyanin. Whenever possible, use wild blueberries because they are higher in antioxidants in a volume-to-volume comparison with cultivated berries.

PER SERVING Calories: 102; Carbohydrates: 27g; Glycemic Load: 7; Fiber: 5g; Protein: 1g; Sodium: 2mg; Fat: 0g

Walnut Baked Pears

5-Ingredient, Dairy-Free, Fertility Boost, Inflammation Fighter

Serves 4 Dried fruit is usually packed with preservatives and sugar, which makes it inappropriate for diets meant to reduce or prevent insulin resistance. Dried cherries are naturally sweet and do not need added sweeteners, and moderation is key. Look for organic and sugar-free options. Cherries are antioxidant rich and a source of melatonin, a naturally occurring hormone that regulates sleep patterns. Sleep is important to general good health and for reducing the effect of PCOS.

PREP: 15 minutes
COOK: 20 minutes

4 pears, cored, left whole

1 cup chopped walnuts

¼ cup dried cherries

2 tablespoons almond butter

2 tablespoons rolled oats

¼ teaspoon ground cinnamon

1. Preheat the oven to 400°F.

2. Stand the pears in an 8-by-8-inch baking dish.

3. In a small bowl, stir together the walnuts, cherries, almond butter, oats, and cinnamon until well combined. Spoon the filling into the center of the pears.

4. Bake for about 20 minutes, until the fruit is tender.

LOWER CALORIE TIP Reduce the walnuts to ½ cup and increase the oats to ½ cup to cut 50 calories and 8 grams of fat from the dish. This change will also increase the protein by 1 gram per serving.

PER SERVING Calories: 360; Carbohydrates: 33g; Glycemic Load: 8; Fiber: 8g; Protein: 7g; Sodium: 8mg; Fat: 22g

Lemon Curd with Blueberries

5-Ingredient, Dairy-Free, Fertility Boost, Gluten-Free, Inflammation Fighter, Lower Calorie

Serves 4 This sunny, tart dessert is packed with antioxidants and makes a good choice for breakfast if you add a sprinkle of homemade Pecan Coconut Granola (page 54). Berries, honey, lemon juice, coconut oil, and egg yolks all support fertility. Vanilla is also an antioxidant, containing vanillic acid and vanillin, which can protect against liver inflammation. Vanilla can also help lower cholesterol and help support weight-loss goals.

PREP: 10 minutes, plus chilling time
COOK: 5 minutes

4 large egg yolks

2 tablespoons raw honey

¼ cup melted coconut oil

Zest and juice of 1 lemon

1 teaspoon pure vanilla extract

Pinch sea salt

2 cups fresh blueberries

1. In a medium saucepan over medium heat, combine the egg yolks, honey, coconut oil, lemon zest and juice, vanilla, and salt. Cook for about 5 minutes, whisking constantly, until the curd thickens.

2. Pass the curd through a sieve into a bowl. Cover the bowl with plastic wrap, pressing it down onto the surface of the curd. Refrigerate the curd until cold.

3. Serve spooned over the blueberries.

INFLAMMATION FIGHTER TIP Blueberries are extremely high in antioxidants, especially anthocyanins, which can turn off immune and inflammatory genes. Blueberries are also a stellar source of resveratrol, a polyphenol that helps reduce free radicals in the body. Eat at least ½ cup of blueberries several times a week to benefit from their effects.

PER SERVING Calories: 249; Carbohydrates: 20g; Glycemic Load: 7; Fiber: 2g; Protein: 3g; Sodium: 9mg; Fat: 18g

Raspberry Plum Crumble

5-Ingredient, 30-Minute, Dairy-Free, Fertility Boost, Inflammation Fighter, Lower Calorie

Serves 6 Chia seeds might seem like an odd filling choice for a sweet fruit dessert, but they soak up the juices seeping from the raspberries and plums while the fruit cooks, creating a thick, luscious texture. Chia seeds are incredibly rich in omega-3 fatty acids, even more than salmon by volume. Walnuts are also packed with omega-3s, and there is about 120 percent of the recommended daily amount in a serving of this crumble. Omega-3 fatty acid is the most potent anti-inflammatory compound you can eat.

PREP: 10 minutes
COOK: 20 minutes

2 cups fresh raspberries
2 plums, pitted and chopped
3 tablespoons chia seeds
1 tablespoon raw honey
1 cup rolled oats
1 cup ground walnuts
¼ cup coconut oil
1 teaspoon ground cinnamon

1. Preheat the oven to 400°F.

2. In a medium bowl, toss together the raspberries, plums, chia seeds, and honey. Transfer the fruit mixture to an 8-by-8-inch baking dish.

3. In a small bowl, toss together the oats, walnuts, coconut oil, and cinnamon until it resembles coarse crumbs. Sprinkle the oat mixture over the fruit.

4. Bake for about 20 minutes, until the fruit is bubbly and the topping is golden brown.

FERTILITY BOOST TIP Although plums are delicious, especially in summer when they are sweet and fragrant, doubling the berries can support healthy hormone levels and prevent cellular damage to ova. Blueberries, cranberries, strawberries, and blackberries are all delicious in this tempting dessert.

PER SERVING Calories: 265; Carbohydrates: 30g; Glycemic Load: 11; Fiber: 8g; Protein: 7g; Sodium: 2mg; Fat: 14g

9

Broths, Sauces, and Dressings

Fiery Peanut Sauce

30-Minute, Dairy-Free, Fertility Boost, Gluten-Free, Lower Calorie

Makes 1½ cups Peanut sauce is traditionally served with chicken satay (skewers) in Indonesian cuisine, but it can be delicious with other ingredients, such as pork, fish, and vegetables. If you like your food very spicy, increase the red pepper flakes, which will also increase the inflammation-fighting capsaicin. Capsaicin aids with weight loss because that lovely heat you feel takes energy to produce and burns calories. Also, a meal that includes dried chile peppers requires less insulin to lower blood sugar.

PREP: 10 minutes
COOK: none

½ cup natural peanut butter

½ cup coconut milk

2 teaspoons coconut aminos

1 teaspoon minced garlic

Zest and juice of 1 lime

1 teaspoon chopped fresh cilantro leaves

Pinch red pepper flakes

In a small bowl, whisk together all the ingredients. Refrigerate the sauce in a sealed container for up to 1 week.

FERTILITY BOOST TIP Peanut butter is a fantastic source of iron, an important mineral because low levels of iron have been linked to infertility. Plant sources of iron (nonheme iron) are considered the best choice for women trying to conceive, so include peanut butter and other sources, such as bok choy, cashews, dark leafy greens, quinoa, sunflower seeds, and tahini, in your diet frequently.

PER SERVING (2 tablespoons) Calories: 83; Carbohydrates: 3g; Glycemic Load: 0; Fiber: 1g; Protein: 3g; Sodium: 59mg; Fat: 7g

Fresh Chile Pesto

30-Minute, Dairy-Free, Fertility Boost, Gluten-Free, Inflammation Fighter, Lower Calorie

Makes 1 cup Chiles are a superlative choice for women with PCOS because they boost fertility and fight inflammation. Chiles can increase blood flow so reproductive organs remain healthy. They stimulate endorphin production, which helps the body deal better with fertility-limiting stress. Chiles are also high in vitamin C, sinapic acid, and ferulic acid, all of which help reduce inflammation. Toss with zucchini noodles, spread on fish or poultry, or serve as a dip for celery and carrots sticks.

PREP: 5 minutes
COOK: 18 minutes

1 teaspoon extra-virgin olive oil

¼ cup chopped sweet onion

1 teaspoon minced garlic

½ cup water

¼ cup slivered almonds

3 dried chiles of choice, chopped

½ teaspoon ground cumin

¼ teaspoon ground coriander

1. In a medium skillet over medium-high heat, heat the olive oil.

2. Add the onion and garlic and sauté for about 3 minutes, until softened.

3. Stir in the water, almonds, chiles, cumin, and coriander. Bring the mixture to a boil. Reduce the heat to low and simmer for about 15 minutes, until the chiles soften. Transfer the mixture to a blender and pulse until smooth.

4. Refrigerate the pesto in a sealed container for up to 1 week.

INGREDIENT TIP This recipe is called "fresh" chile pesto even though it uses dried peppers. The chiles reconstitute in the simmering water to create a more intensely flavored sauce than if you used fresh produce.

PER SERVING (1 tablespoon) Calories: 17; Carbohydrates: 1g; Glycemic Load: 0; Fiber: 0g; Protein: 1g; Sodium: 1mg; Fat: 1g

Sesame-Orange Stir-Fry Sauce

30-Minute, Dairy-Free, Fertility Boost, Gluten-Free, Lower Calorie

Makes 1 cup Citrus juice, sesame oil, and sesame seeds blend to create a stir-fry sauce that can be used for any dish—vegetarian, pork, chicken, beef, and shrimp. Oranges, both the juice and the zest, contain a staggering amount of anti-inflammatory components—170 different phytonutrients—and more than 60 flavonoids. Oranges are high in a compound called myo-inositol, which can help balance blood sugar and improve egg quality and the follicular environment.

PREP: 5 minutes
COOK: none

½ cup freshly squeezed orange juice

¼ cup low-sodium chicken broth

2 tablespoons coconut aminos

1 tablespoon sesame oil

1 tablespoon orange zest

1 tablespoon arrowroot powder

1 tablespoon sesame seeds

1. In a small bowl, whisk together all the ingredients.

2. Refrigerate the sauce in a sealed container for up to 1 week.

FERTILITY BOOST TIP Increase the sesame seeds to 2 tablespoons to double the amount of healthy omega-3 fatty acids in this sweet sauce. Sesame seeds can also decrease inflammation that can disrupt hormone levels in the body.

PER SERVING (2 tablespoons) Calories: 48; Carbohydrates: 4g; Glycemic Load: 1; Fiber: 1g; Protein: 1g; Sodium: 152mg; Fat: 3g

Tomato Dressing

5-Ingredient, 30-Minute, Dairy-Free, Gluten-Free, Inflammation Fighter, Lower Calorie

Makes 1 cup Salads are a staple for people trying to lose weight and follow a healthier lifestyle, and this flavorful dressing can transform a basic salad into an exceptional meal. Sun-dried tomatoes are rich in flavor and high in fiber, vitamins A, B, and C, calcium, zinc, and protein. You can easily make your own sun-dried tomatoes: Halve plum tomatoes and dry them in a low-heat oven (about 275°F) for about 4 hours, or until they reach your desired texture.

PREP: 15 minutes
COOK: none

6 sun-dried tomatoes

3 tablespoons balsamic vinegar

1 tablespoon minced fresh basil leaves

2 teaspoons minced garlic

½ cup extra-virgin olive oil

Sea salt, for seasoning

Freshly ground black pepper, for seasoning

1. In a blender, combine the tomatoes, vinegar, basil, and garlic. Pulse until smooth. Transfer the mixture to a small bowl.

2. Whisk in the olive oil. Season the dressing with salt and pepper.

3. Refrigerate the dressing in a sealed container for up to 1 week.

INFLAMMATION FIGHTER TIP Balsamic vinegar contains powerful antioxidants called polyphenols, which can boost the immune system and fight cell damage. Including this delightful ingredient regularly in your diet—as little as 1 tablespoon—can increase insulin sensitivity.

PER SERVING (2 tablespoons) Calories: 130; Carbohydrates: 2g; Glycemic Load: 1; Fiber: 0g; Protein: 0g; Sodium: 33mg; Fat: 14g

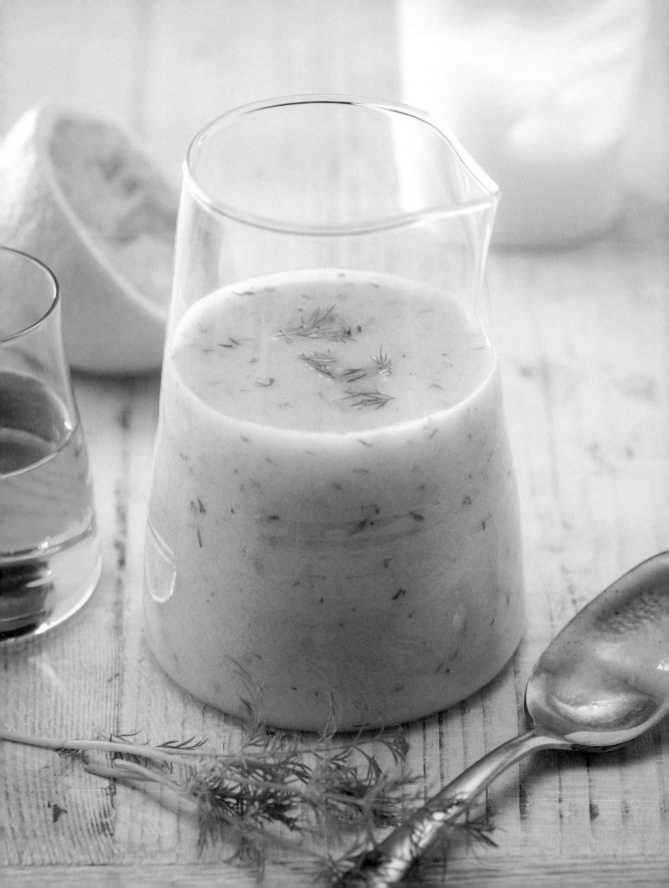

Dijon-Lemon Marinade

5-Ingredient, 30-Minute, Dairy-Free, Gluten-Free, Lower Calorie

Makes ½ cup Honey and mustard are commonly used in vinaigrettes because the sweet and sour mix stimulates the taste buds. The lemon juice brightens the flavor and can prevent oxidization of certain ingredients in your salads, like avocado, apple, or pear. Mustard was actually the traditional symbol of fertility for ancient Hindus and is high in omega-3 fatty acids, selenium, and manganese, which all encourage healthy fertility. Double or triple this recipe so you always have a perfect dressing ready for tossing salads, drizzling on baked fish, or marinating meat and poultry.

PREP: 5 minutes
COOK: none

¼ cup extra-virgin olive oil

2 tablespoons freshly squeezed lemon juice

1 tablespoon Dijon mustard

1 teaspoon raw honey

1 tablespoon chopped fresh dill

Sea salt, for seasoning

Freshly ground black pepper, for seasoning

1. In a small bowl, whisk the olive oil, lemon juice, mustard, honey, and dill until emulsified. Season the dressing with salt and pepper.

2. Refrigerate the dressing in a sealed container for up to 2 weeks.

COOKING TIP Store the dressing in a pretty bottle and give it a vigorous shake before using.

PER SERVING (1 tablespoon) Calories: 64; Carbohydrates: 1g; Glycemic Load: 0; Fiber: 0g; Protein: 0g; Sodium: 21mg; Fat: 7g

Inflammation-Busting Broth

Dairy-Free, Gluten-Free, Inflammation Fighter, Lower Calorie

Makes 8 cups You can buy good-quality chicken broth because many companies are making it their business to support the health industry, which demands less sodium and fat in most cases. Making your own broth, though, allows you to add ingredients you want, including the apple cider vinegar that creates such a mineral- and vitamin-packed liquid. Make a couple of batches of this broth and store them for your recipe needs. Comfort and inflammation-busting power in one delicious cup.

PREP: 15 minutes
COOK: 2 hours

1½ pounds chicken bones

4 celery stalks, roughly chopped

4 garlic cloves, crushed

2 carrots, cut into 1-inch pieces

1 sweet onion, cut into eighths

1 tablespoon apple cider vinegar

4 fresh parsley sprigs

2 bay leaves

10 cups water

1. In a large stockpot, combine the chicken bones, celery, garlic, carrots, onion, vinegar, parsley, bay leaves, and water.

2. Bring the liquid to a boil. Reduce the heat to low and simmer for 2 hours.

3. Strain the broth through a fine-mesh sieve and cool.

4. Refrigerate the broth in sealed containers for up to 1 week, or freeze for up to 1 month.

INFLAMMATION FIGHTER TIP The apple cider vinegar in this broth adds powerful anti-inflammatory punch and it draws out the nutrients from the bones. The onion and garlic also add to the health effects of the broth, so feel free to add more of these ingredients.

PER SERVING (1 cup) Calories: 54; Carbohydrates: 0g; Glycemic Load: 2; Fiber: 0g; Protein: 5g; Sodium: 45mg; Fat: 1g

Simple Vegetable Broth

Dairy-Free, Gluten-Free, Lower Calorie

Makes 12 cups Most of the flavor in this soothing vegetable broth comes from the celery, especially the greens—so be sure to include the full amount in the recipe. Celery has great anti-inflammatory properties because it contains phytonutrients and many antioxidants. It is also a good source of vitamin C, beta-carotene, and manganese. These elements help decrease oxidative damage to the body. Celery and greens are also high in calcium, magnesium, and phosphorus.

PREP: 15 minutes
COOK: 1 hour

4 celery stalks with greens, roughly chopped

3 carrots, roughly chopped

1 sweet onion, cut into eighths

3 garlic cloves, crushed

6 fresh thyme sprigs

3 fresh parsley sprigs

2 bay leaves

1 teaspoon peppercorns

4 quarts water

1. In a large stockpot over high heat, combine the celery, carrots, onion, garlic, thyme, parsley, bay leaves, peppercorns, and water.

2. Bring the broth to a boil. Reduce the heat and simmer for 1 hour.

3. Strain the broth through a fine-mesh sieve and cool.

4. Refrigerate the broth in sealed containers for up to 1 week, or freeze for up to 1 month.

COOKING TIP The best part of making your own vegetable broth is that you can use carrot peels, onion ends, and any type of vegetables or herbs in your refrigerator. Just simmer, strain, and store.

PER SERVING (1 cup) Calories: 12; Carbohydrates: 3g; Glycemic Load: 0; Fiber: 0g; Protein: 0g; Sodium: 34mg; Fat: 0g

Quick Marinara Sauce

5-Ingredient, Dairy-Free, Gluten-Free, Inflammation Fighter, Lower Calorie

Serves 4 A good flavorful marinara sauce is a culinary masterpiece, and some of the best sauces are created using good-quality, yet minimal, ingredients. For the freshest flavor, look for sun-ripened heirloom tomatoes, in any color, even though they can look strange. Tomatoes are rich in vitamins C and K as well as lycopene, and heirloom varieties have even higher levels of these nutrients because they are grown organically.

PREP: 10 minutes
COOK: 25 minutes

2 tablespoons extra-virgin olive oil

1 sweet onion, chopped

2 teaspoons minced garlic

4 cups diced tomatoes

2 tablespoons chopped fresh oregano leaves

1 tablespoon chopped fresh basil leaves

Sea salt, for seasoning

Freshly ground black pepper, for seasoning

1. In a large saucepan over medium-high heat, heat the olive oil.

2. Add the onion and garlic and sauté for about 3 minutes, until softened.

3. Stir in the tomatoes, oregano, and basil. Bring the sauce to a boil. Reduce the heat to low and simmer for 20 minutes.

4. Season the sauce with salt and pepper.

INGREDIENT TIP To save time, use good-quality sodium-free canned diced tomatoes instead of fresh. You will notice the color of the sauce will be darker and richer with canned products.

PER SERVING Calories: 105; Carbohydrates: 10g; Glycemic Load: 4; Fiber: 3g; Protein: 2g; Sodium: 10mg; Fat: 7g

Spiced Cherry Sauce

30-Minute, Dairy-Free, Gluten-Free, Inflammation Fighter, Lower Calorie

Makes 2 cups This bright sauce can be used in many ways, such as spooned over broiled fish or barbecued chicken, or as a tempting dip for vegetables or fruit. The ginger and jalapeño pepper add a hefty kick of heat that blends beautifully with the sweet cherries. If fresh cherries are not available, you can use flash-frozen cherries because their nutritional value is not affected by the freezing process.

PREP: 10 minutes
COOK: none

2 cups fresh cherries, pitted and coarsely diced

½ jalapeño pepper, chopped

Zest and juice of 1 lemon

2 teaspoons grated fresh ginger

½ teaspoon ground cumin

¼ teaspoon ground coriander

1. In a blender, combine the cherries, jalapeño, lemon zest and juice, ginger, cumin, and coriander. Pulse until very smooth. If the sauce is too thick, add some water to reach the right consistency.

2. Refrigerate the sauce in a sealed container for up to 1 week.

> **INFLAMMATION FIGHTER TIP** Ginger creates a complex heat when combined with the fresh jalapeño in this sauce. Ginger is considered to have antioxidant, anti-inflammatory, and antibacterial characteristics because it contains compounds called gingerols, which block enzymes and genes that can create inflammation in the body. Include this potent rhizome in your recipes whenever appropriate.

PER SERVING (¼ cup) Calories: 22; Carbohydrates: 6g; Glycemic Load: 2; Fiber: 1g; Protein: 0g; Sodium: 0mg; Fat: 0g

Garlic-Herb Marinade

5-Ingredient, 30-Minute, Dairy-Free, Gluten-Free, Inflammation Fighter, Lower Calorie

Makes 1 cup Fats are often seen as bad, but good unsaturated fats, such as in extra-virgin olive oil, support healthy fertility. Make sure to use extra-virgin olive oil because other pressings do not reduce the inflammation markers like extra-virgin does. The phytonutrient levels in this oil are considerably higher than other types. Extra-virgin olive oil is extremely high in omega-3 fatty acids because oleic acid makes up 70 to 85 percent of its fat. Use this versatile marinade for meat, poultry, fish—or pretty much anything you want to marinate.

PREP: 15 minutes
COOK: none

½ cup extra-virgin olive oil

Zest and juice of 1 lemon

1 tablespoon apple cider vinegar

2 teaspoons minced garlic

1 tablespoon chopped fresh thyme leaves

1 teaspoon chopped fresh rosemary leaves

Sea salt, for seasoning

Freshly ground black pepper, for seasoning

1. In a small bowl, whisk the olive oil, lemon zest and juice, vinegar, garlic, thyme, and rosemary until well combined. Season the marinade with salt and pepper.

2. Refrigerate the marinade in a sealed container for up to 1 week.

INFLAMMATION FIGHTER TIP Apple cider vinegar is valued as a medicinal ingredient for helping many ailments, including those caused by inflammation. It helps balance blood sugar and is very high in vitamin C. To boost inflammation-fighting benefits, omit the lemon juice in this marinade and use 2 extra tablespoons apple cider vinegar inistead.

PER SERVING (2 tablespoons) Calories: 122; Carbohydrates: 1g; Glycemic Load: 0; Fiber: 0g; Protein: 0g; Sodium: 1mg; Fat: 14g

Jerk Marinade

30-Minute, Dairy-Free, Fertility Boost, Gluten-Free, Inflammation Fighter, Lower Calorie

Makes 1 cup "Jerk" refers to grilled or broiled meats in a fiery sweet sauce, and this marinade is a simpler version of the complex mixtures created in South America. Spices and ingredients such as jalapeno peppers are potent anti-inflammatories, and the cinnamon can help control blood sugar levels. Use this marinade with lean proteins such as chicken breast and pork to boost fertility.

PREP: 10 minutes
COOK: none

1 sweet onion,
finely chopped

1 jalapeño pepper,
finely chopped

2 tablespoons
coconut aminos

1 tablespoon extra-virgin
olive oil

1 tablespoon apple
cider vinegar

1 tablespoon raw honey

2 teaspoons chopped
fresh thyme

1 teaspoon paprika

1 teaspoon ground cinnamon

½ teaspoon freshly ground
black pepper

½ teaspoon ground nutmeg

¼ teaspoon sea salt

1. Place the onion, jalapeño pepper, coconut aminos, olive oil, cider vinegar, thyme, honey, paprika, cinnamon, black pepper, nutmeg, and sea salt in a blender and pulse until smooth.

2. Store in the refrigerator for up to one week in a sealed container.

INGREDIENT TIP Jalapeño peppers come in a range of hotness from mild to quite fiery, getting hotter as they age. If you want a hotter pepper for this marinade, look for one with striations on the skin, little white lines, and white flecks.

PER SERVING (1 tablespoon) Calories: 14; Carbohydrates: 2g; Glycemic Load: 1; Fiber: 0g; Protein: 0g; Sodium: 99mg; Fat: 1g

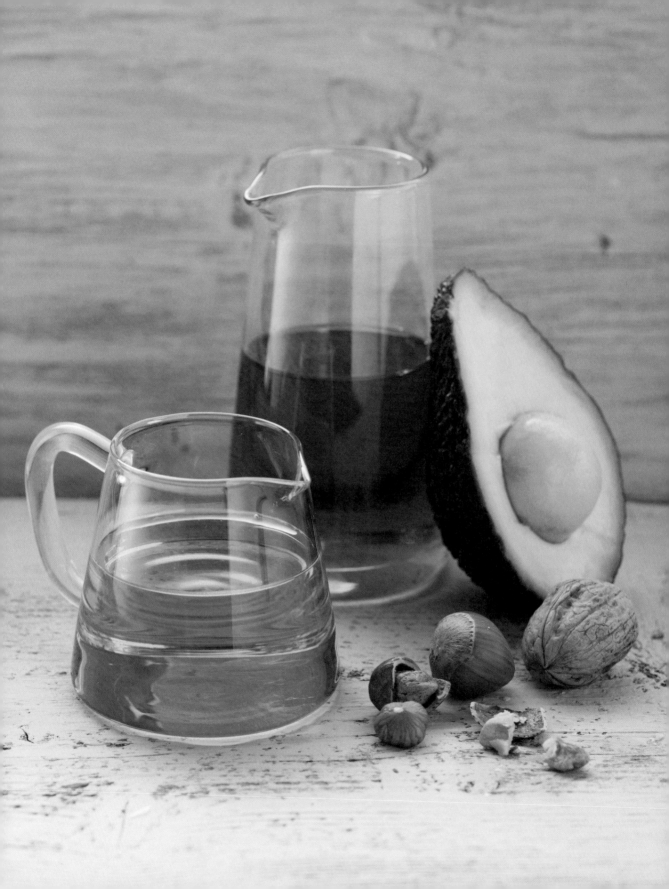

Acknowledgments

I would like to thank my friends and family for sticking by me during the tumultuous time of my PCOS diagnosis. I am blessed with a great number of positive, healthy role models in my life who were willing to guide me through my own journey of healing.

I am also grateful to myself, for having the courage and persistence—even during the toughest and most painful periods—to pursue health and vitality.

Thank you to all of my clients who have trusted me with their hormonal health and taught me even more about my own condition by sharing their private experiences and sufferings with me.

Finally, thank you to the entire team at Callisto Media, who are always a pleasure to work with.

Resources

The following additional resources provide more information about PCOS, insulin resistance, self-compassion, and positive body image.

A Couple's Guide to PCOS

www.couplesguidetopcos.com

An online video course designed to help couples maintain a strong relationship while dealing with PCOS. Whether your goal is to become pregnant, lose weight, or feel healthy overall while growing old together, this course can help.

American Psychological Association (APA) Help Center

www.apa.org/helpcenter /choose-therapist.aspx

Provides a list of qualified therapists in your area, broken down by expertise and level. Therapy can help you uncover and overcome any psychological barriers preventing you from achieving full health and wellness.

Center for Young Women's Health

youngwomenshealth.org/2012/05/30 /self-esteem/

For younger women who struggle with poor self-esteem and body image. The website also contains resources for PCOS sufferers.

Infertility Network

www.infertilitynetwork.org

A charity that provides information and support for women worldwide who have trouble conceiving.

Intuitive Eating

www.intuitiveeating.com

Offers instructions for beginning an intuitive eating process and eating more mindfully.

National Institute of Diabetes and Digestive and Kidney Diseases

www.niddk.nih.gov/health-information /health-topics/Diabetes/insulin -resistance-prediabetes

Explains how insulin resistance and pre-diabetes develop. For those who would like to gain a better scientific understanding of the condition.

Natural Fertility Info

www.natural-fertility-info.com /pcos-fertility-diet

Contains a comprehensive list of what supplements can help improve PCOS, and why.

PCOS Awareness Association

www.pcosaa.org

A nonprofit organization that aims to spread awareness about PCOS by increasing early diagnosis rates and overcoming the various individual symptoms of the condition. It links to a number of support groups worldwide.

PCOS Diet Support Group

www.facebook.com/PCOSDietSupport/

A community of women affected by PCOS. Within this Facebook group, the women share articles, general tips, and positive mantras to help each other overcome their PCOS.

PCOS Support Group

www.pcos.supportgroups.com

An active community with almost 20,000 members who suffer from PCOS.

Resolve

www.resolve.org

A nonprofit organization that works to improve the lives of men and women dealing with infertility. It offers support groups for couples going through infertility treatments.

Society for Reproductive Endocrinology and Infertility

www.socrei.org

Provides the latest research and information about infertility, and connects the public with the best hormonal specialists.

The Insulin Resistance Diet for PCOS

A book I wrote in 2016 that provides further details about the development of PCOS and how to manage it through a four-week diet plan and lifestyle changes. It is a great sister book for this plan.

The National Eating Disorders Association

www.nationaleatingdisorders.org /developing-and-maintaining-positive -body-image

A nonprofit organization for those who are affected by eating disorders. It features a great amount of information for building a healthy body image.

References

Adams, P. "The Impact of Brief High-Intensity Exercise on Blood Glucose Levels." *Journal of Diabetes, Metabolic Syndrome, and Obesity: Targets and Therapy* 6, no. 1 (February 2013): 113–122. doi:10.2147/DMSO.S29222.

American Heart Association. "Managing Blood Pressure with a Heart-Healthy Diet." Last modified December 12, 2016. Accessed February 4, 2017. www.heart.org/HEARTORG /Conditions/HighBloodPressure /MakeChangesThatMatter/Managing-Blood -Pressure-with-a-Heart-Healthy-Diet _UCM_301879_Article.jsp#.WOlNSojytnII

Biaggioni, I., and S. Davis. "Caffeine: A Cause of Insulin Resistance?" *Diabetes Care* 25, no. 2 (February 2002): 399–400. doi:10.2337/diacare.25.2.399.

Bloomgarden, Z. "Topics in Type 2 Diabetes and Insulin Resistance." *Diabetes Care* 32, no. 2 (February 2009): 13–19.

Collins, G., and B. Rossi. "The Impact of Lifestyle Modifications, Diet, and Vitamin Supplementation on Natural Fertility." *Fertility Research and Practice* 1, no. 11 (July 2015). doi:10.1186/s40738-015-0003-4.

Corbould, A. "Effects of Androgens on Insulin Action in Women: Is Androgen Excess a Component of Female Metabolic Syndrome?" *Diabetes Metabolism Research and Reviews* 24, no. 7 (October 2008): 520–532. doi:10.1002/dmrr.872.

Ferin, M. "Stress and the Reproductive Cycle." *The Journal of Clinical Endocrinology and Metabolism* 84, no. 6 (June 1999): 1768–1774. doi.org/10.1210/jcem.84.6.5367.

Gudmundsdottir, S., W. Flanders, and L. Augestad. "Physical Activity and Fertility in Women: The North-Trøndelag Health Study." *Human Reproduction* 24, no. 12 (December 2009): 3196–3204. doi:10.1093/humrep/dep337.

Health Line. "Testosterone Levels by Age." Last modified March 23, 2015. Accessed February 2, 2017. www.healthline.com /health/low-testosterone/testosterone -levels-by-age.

Hutchinson, S., N. Stepto, C. Harrison, L. Moran, B. Strauss, and H. Teede. "Effects of Exercise on Insulin Resistance and Body Composition in Overweight and Obese Women with and without Polycystic Ovary Syndrome." *The Journal of Clinical Endocrinology and Metabolism* 96, no. 1 (January 2011): E48–56. doi:10.1210 /jc.2010-0828.

Kiddy, D., D. Hamilton-Fairley, A. Bush, F. Short, V. Anyaoku, M. Reed, and S. Franks. "Improvement in Endocrine and Ovarian Function during Dietary Treatment of Obese Women with Polycystic Ovary Syndrome." *Clinical Endocrinology* (Oxford) 36, no. 1 (January 1992): 105–111.

Knutson, K. "Impact of Sleep and Sleep Loss on Glucose Homeostasis and Appetite Regulation." *Sleep Medicine Clinics* 2, no. 2 (June 2007): 187–197. doi:10.1016/j.jsmc.2007.03.004.

Kondracki, N. "The Link between Sleep and Weight Gain–Research Shows Poor Sleep Quality Raises Obesity and Chronic Disease Risk." *Today's Dietitian* 14, no. 6 (June 2012): 48.

Kresser, C. "How Inflammation Makes You Fat and Diabetic (and Vice Versa)." Last modified September 15, 2010. Accessed February 5, 2017. www.chriskresser.com /how-inflammation-makes-you-fat-and -diabetic-and-vice-versa.

National Institute of Diabetes and Digestive and Kidney Diseases. "Prediabetes and Insulin Resistance." Accessed January 28, 2017. www.niddk.nih.gov/health-information /diabetes/overview/what-is-diabetes/ prediabetes-insulin-resistance.

Natural Fertility Info. "How to Reduce the Damaging Effects of PCOS on Fertility through Diet and Herbs." Accessed February 12, 2016. www.natural-fertility-info.com /pcos-fertility-diet.

Norman, R., M. Noakes, R. Wu, M. Davies, L. Moran, and J. Wang. "Improving Reproductive Performance in Overweight /Obese Women with Effective Weight Management." *Human Reproductive Update* 10, no. 3 (May 2004): 267–280. doi:10.1093/humupd/dmh018.

O'Neill, H. "AMPK and Exercise: Glucose Uptake and Insulin Sensitivity." *The Diabetes and Metabolism Journal* 37, no. 1 (February 2013): 1–21. doi:10.4093 /dmj.2013.37.1.1.

Paddon-Jones, D., E. Westman, R. Mattes, R. Wolfe, A. Astrup, and M. Westerterp-Plantenga. "Protein, Weight Management, and Satiety." *The American Journal of Clinical Nutrition* 87, no. 5 (May 2008): 1558S–1561S.

Ranabir, S., and K. Reetu. "Stress and Hormones." *Indian Journal of Endocrinology and Metabolism* 15, no. 1 (January 2011): 18–22. doi:10.4103/2230-8210.77573.

Resolve. "Fast Facts about Infertility." Last modified April 19, 2015. Accessed February 6, 2017. www.resolve.org/about /fast-facts-about-fertility.html.

Stepto, N., S. Cassar, A. Joham, S. Hutchinson, C. Harrison, R. Goldstein, and H. Teede. "Women with Polycystic Ovary Syndrome Have Intrinsic Insulin Resistance on Euglycaemic-Hyperinsulaemic Clamp." *Human Reproduction* 28, no. 3 (March 2013): 777–784. doi.org/10.1093/humrep /des463.

Traub, M. "Assessing and Treating Insulin Resistance in Women with Polycystic Ovarian Syndrome." *World Journal of Diabetes* 2, no. 3 (March 2011): 33–40. doi:10.4239/wjd .v2.i3.33.

Glycemic Index and Glycemic Load Food List

The following is a list of the glycemic index and glycemic load rankings of many common carbohydrates. Foods are ranked between 0 and 100 based on how they affect one's blood glucose level. The best choices are foods that range between 55 to 69 on the glycemic index.

Remember that it is more important to pay attention to the glycemic load of a food–that is, the amount of carbohydrates it contains per serving. The best choices have low (less than 10) or moderate (between 10 and 20) glycemic loads.

FOOD	GLYCEMIC INDEX	SERVING SIZE grams, unless noted othewise	GLYCEMIC LOAD per serving
Bakery Products			
Bagel, white	72	70	25
Baguette, white	95	30	15
Barley bread	34	30	7
Corn tortilla	52	50	12
Croissant	67	57	17
Doughnut	76	47	17
Pita bread	68	30	10
Sourdough rye	48	30	6
Soya and linseed bread	36	30	3
Sponge cake	46	63	17
Wheat tortilla	30	50	8
White wheat flour bread	71	30	10
Whole-wheat bread	71	30	9

FOOD	GLYCEMIC INDEX	SERVING SIZE grams unless noted otherwise	GLYCEMIC LOAD per serving
Beverages			
Apple juice, unsweetened	44	250 mL	30
Coca-Cola	63	250 mL	16
Gatorade	78	250 mL	12
Lucozade	95	250 mL	40
Orange juice, unsweetened	50	250 mL	12
Tomato juice, canned	38	250 mL	4
Breakfast Cereals			
All-Bran	55	30	12
Cocoa Krispies	77	30	20
Cornflakes	93	30	23
Muesli, average	66	30	16
Oatmeal, average	55	50	13
Special K	69	30	14
Dairy			
Ice cream, regular	57	50	6
Milk, full-fat	41	250 mL	5
Milk, skim	32	250 mL	4
Reduced-fat yogurt with fruit	33	200	11
Fruits			
Apple	39	120	6
Banana, ripe	62	120	16

FOOD	GLYCEMIC INDEX	SERVING SIZE *grams unless noted otherwise*	GLYCEMIC LOAD *per serving*
Fruits, continued			
Cherries	22	120	3
Dates, dried	42	60	18
Grapefruit	25	120	3
Grapes	59	120	11
Mango	41	120	8
Orange	40	120	4
Peach	42	120	5
Pear	38	120	4
Pineapple	51	120	8
Raisins	64	60	28
Strawberries	40	120	1
Watermelon	72	120	4
Grains			
Brown Rice	50	150	16
Buckwheat	45	150	13
Bulgur	30	50	11
Corn on the cob	60	150	20
Couscous	65	150	9
Fettuccini, average	32	180	15
Gnocchi	68	180	33
Macaroni, average	47	180	23

FOOD	GLYCEMIC INDEX	SERVING SIZE grams unless noted otherwise	GLYCEMIC LOAD per serving
Grains, continued			
Quinoa	53	150	13
Spaghetti, white	46	180	22
Spaghetti, whole-wheat	42	180	26
Vermicelli noodles	35	180	16
White rice	89	150	43
Legumes			
Baked beans	40	150	6
Black beans	30	150	7
Butter beans	36	150	8
Chickpeas	10	150	3
Kidney beans	29	150	7
Lentils	29	150	5
Navy beans	31	150	9
Soy beans	50	150	1
Snack Foods			
Cashews, salted	27	50	3
Corn chips, plain, salted	42	50	11
Fruit Roll-Ups	99	30	24
Graham crackers	74	25	14
Honey	61	25	12
Hummus	6	30	0

FOOD	GLYCEMIC INDEX	SERVING SIZE grams unless noted otherwise	GLYCEMIC LOAD per serving
Snack foods, continued			
M&M's, peanut	33	30	6
Microwave popcorn, plain	55	20	6
Muesli bar	61	30	13
Nutella	33	20	4
Peanuts	7	50	0
Potato chips, average	51	50	12
Pretzels	83	30	16
Rice cakes	82	25	17
Rye crisps	64	25	11
Shortbread	64	25	10
Vanilla wafers	77	25	14
Walnuts	15	28	0
Vegetables			
Beets	64	80	4
Carrot	35	80	2
Green peas	51	80	4
Parsnip	52	80	4
Sweet potato, average	70	150	22
White potato, boiled	81	150	22
Yam	54	150	20

Sources: Harvard Health Publications (www.health.harvard.edu/healthy-eating/glycemic_index_and _glycemic_load_for_100_foods) and Mendosa.com (www.mendosa.com/gilists.htm).

Conversion Tables

Volume Equivalents (Liquid)

US STANDARD	US STANDARD (OUNCES)	METRIC (APPROXIMATE)
2 tablespoons	1 fl. oz.	30 mL
¼ cup	2 fl. oz.	60 mL
½ cup	4 fl. oz.	120 mL
1 cup	8 fl. oz.	240 mL
1½ cups	12 fl. oz.	355 mL
2 cups or 1 pint	16 fl. oz.	475 mL
4 cups or 1 quart	32 fl. oz.	1 L
1 gallon	128 fl. oz.	4 L

Oven Temperatures

FAHRENHEIT	CELSIUS (APPROXIMATE)
250°F	120°C
300°F	150°C
325°F	165°C
350°F	180°C
375°F	190°C
400°F	200°C
425°F	220°C
450°F	230°C

Volume Equivalents (Dry)

US STANDARD	METRIC (APPROXIMATE)
⅛ teaspoon	0.5 mL
¼ teaspoon	1 mL
½ teaspoon	2 mL
¾ teaspoon	4 mL
1 teaspoon	5 mL
1 tablespoon	15 mL
¼ cup	59 mL
⅓ cup	79 mL
½ cup	118 mL
⅔ cup	156 mL
¾ cup	177 mL
1 cup	235 mL
2 cups or 1 pint	475 mL
3 cups	700 mL
4 cups or 1 quart	1 L

Weight Equivalents

US STANDARD	METRIC (APPROXIMATE)
½ ounce	15 g
1 ounce	30 g
2 ounces	60 g
4 ounces	115 g
8 ounces	225 g
12 ounces	340 g
16 ounces or 1 pound	455 g

The Dirty Dozen and the Clean Fifteen

A nonprofit environmental watchdog organization called Environmental Working Group (EWG) looks at data supplied by the US Department of Agriculture (USDA) and the Food and Drug Administration (FDA) about pesticide residues. Each year it compiles a list of the best and worst pesticide loads found in commercial crops. You can use these lists to decide which fruits and vegetables to buy organic to minimize your exposure to pesticides and which produce is considered safe enough to buy conventionally. This does not mean they are pesticide-free, though, so wash these fruits and vegetables thoroughly.

These lists change every year, so make sure you look up the most recent one before you fill your shopping cart. You'll find the most recent lists, as well as a guide to pesticides in produce, at EWG.org/FoodNews.

Dirty Dozen

Apples	Strawberries
Celery	Sweet bell peppers
Cherries	Tomatoes
Cherry tomatoes	*In addition to the Dirty Dozen, the EWG added two types of produce contaminated with highly toxic organophosphate insecticides:*
Cucumbers	
Grapes	
Nectarines	
Peaches	Kale/Collard greens
Spinach	Hot peppers

Clean Fifteen

Asparagus	Kiwis
Avocados	Mangos
Cabbage	Onions
Cantaloupe	Papayas
Cauliflower	Pineapples
Eggplant	Sweet corn
Grapefruit	Sweet peas (frozen)
Honeydew melon	

Recipe Index

Index

About the Author

As a Fitness-Industry-Education-qualified nutritionist and certified personal trainer, Tara Spencer guides people on their path toward good health. She is experienced with eating disorder recovery, athlete coaching, and utilizing diet as a natural treatment for a number of illnesses. Her work as a nutritionist has given her the opportunity to impact a wide range of people of all ages and stages, from committed and recovering couch potatoes to novice bodybuilding competitors and professional tennis players. She is the author of two previous nutrition books: *The Insulin Resistance Diet Plan and Cookbook*, and *The Migraine Relief Diet*. To learn more about Tara, visit her online at www.sweatlikeapig.com.